LEAVING IT AT THE OFFICE

Leaving It at the Office

A GUIDE TO PSYCHOTHERAPIST SELF-CARE

John C. Norcross
James D. Guy, Jr.

THE GUILFORD PRESS
New York   London

© 2007 John C. Norcross and James D. Guy, Jr.
Published by The Guilford Press
A Division of Guilford Publications, Inc.
72 Spring Street, New York, NY 10012
www.guilford.com

Printed in the United States of America

This book is printed on acid-free paper.

Last digit is print number: 9 8 7 6 5 4 3 2

Library of Congress Cataloging-in-Publication Data

Norcross, John C., 1957–
    Leaving it at the office : a guide to psychotherapist self-care / John C.
Norcross, James D. Guy, Jr.
    p. ; cm.
    Includes bibliographical references and index.
    ISBN-13: 978-1-59385-490-4 (hardcover : alk. paper)
    ISBN-10: 1-59385-490-0 (hardcover : alk. paper)
    ISBN-13: 978-1-59385-576-5 (paperback : alk. paper)
    ISBN-10: 1-59385-576-1 (paperback : alk. paper)
    1. Psychotherapy. 2. Psychotherapists—Mental health. 3. Self-care,
Health.   I. Guy, James D. II. Title.
    [DNLM: 1. Psychotherapy. 2. Attitude of Health Personnel. 3. Burnout,
Professional—prevention & control. 4. Professional—Patient
Relations. 5. Self Care—psychology. WM 62 N827L 2007]
    RC480.8.L4388 2007
    616.89′14—dc22

                                                          2007008155

To our children
(Rebecca, Jonathon, Lisa, Julie, Jonathan, and William)
and to children-at-heart everywhere

About the Authors

John C. Norcross, PhD, ABPP, received his baccalaureate from Rutgers University, earned his master's and doctorate in clinical psychology from the University of Rhode Island, and completed his internship at the Brown University School of Medicine. He is Professor of Psychology and Distinguished University Fellow at the University of Scranton and a clinical psychologist in part-time practice. Author of more than 250 scholarly publications, Dr. Norcross has written or coedited 15 books, the most recent being *Evidence-Based Practices in Mental Health, Psychotherapy Relationships That Work, Authoritative Guide to Self-Help Resources in Mental Health, Psychologists' Desk Reference,* and *Insider's Guide to Graduate Programs in Clinical and Counseling Psychology.* He is past president of the International Society of Clinical Psychology, past president of the American Psychological Association (APA) Division of Psychotherapy, and Council Representative of the APA. Dr. Norcross is also editor of *Journal of Clinical Psychology: In Session* and has been on the editorial boards of a dozen journals. He has received many professional awards, such as the Distinguished Career Contributions to Education and Training Award from the APA, Pennsylvania Professor of the Year from the Carnegie Foundation, the Rosalee Weiss Award from the American Psychological Foundation, and election to the National Academies of Practice. He has given lectures and workshops in 25 countries. Dr. Norcross lives in northeast Pennsylvania with his wife and two children.

James D. Guy, Jr., PhD, ABPP, received his baccalaureate from Wheaton College and his master's of theology and doctorate in clinical psychology from Fuller Theological Seminary. He completed a predoctoral internship at Milwaukee County Mental Health Complex and a postdoctoral fellowship at Northwestern University Institute of Psychiatry. Dr. Guy was Dean and Professor of Psychology at the Graduate School of Psychology at Fuller Theological Seminary from 1995 to 2001. He is currently President and Executive Director of the Headington Institute, a nonprofit organization that provides psychological and spiritual support to humanitarian aid and disaster relief personnel worldwide. He also maintains a private practice in clinical psychology in Pasadena, California. Dr. Guy is a diplomate of the American Board of Professional Psychology and a Fellow of the Divisions of Clinical Psychology and Independent Practice of the American Psychological Association. He has authored numerous articles and monographs on the interface between the professional life and personal relationships of the psychotherapist, including the book *The Personal Life of the Psychotherapist*. He resides in South Pasadena, California, with his wife and four children.

Preface

Leaving It at the Office is a practical synthesis of research literature, clinical wisdom, and therapist experience on, as our subtitle states, psychotherapist self-care. Our principal goals in this book are threefold: first, to remind busy practitioners of the personal and professional need to tend to their own psychological health; second, to provide evidence-based methods for practitioners to nourish themselves; and third, to generate a positive message of self-renewal and growth.

This volume is a curious mix of a "how to," "you should," and, paradoxically, "chill out" manual. The "how to" reflects our practical self-care orientation—how to leave distress at the office and how to grow and refresh yourself. To this end, each chapter concludes with a Self-Care Checklist. The "you should" is our frequent explication of the compelling research and experience that you should replenish yourself, in whatever form or variety succeeds for you, because it enhances you as a person and as a professional. The paradoxical "chill out" is that we do not provide a set of universal prescriptions for self-care nor demand that you partake in specific activities. As psychotherapists (and as people), we are inundated with the tyranny of the shoulds. Our ardent hope is that our book will gently, collegially remind you that our lives are works in progress and that you can practice self-care wholeheartedly, bringing your self fresh to each moment, each patient, and each day.

Self-care is a personal challenge and professional imperative that every psychotherapist—literally, every one—must consciously confront. In other words, our book is intended for all current and future psychotherapists.

We envision *Leaving It at the Office* being read, first of all, by psycho-therapy practitioners of diverse orientations and professions who seek guidance in their own self-care and who believe the personhood of the psychotherapist is one locale for improving our craft. We envision this volume serving, second of all, as a supplemental text in psychotherapy and counseling courses. The book will fit easily into theory, practice, ethics, and professional preparation courses. Like-minded professors may assign our text as part of a graduate seminar on the person of the therapist.

A GOOD BOOK, LIKE A GOOD PSYCHOTHERAPIST

In the mid-1950s Holt and Luborsky (1958) compiled expert opinions on the personal qualities sought in successful applicants for psychotherapy training. Their three criteria pertain equally, it seems to us, to a good book about psychotherapy.

First on the list is an *introspective orientation*: observing inner life, committing to self-observation, engaging in appropriate self-disclosure. Introspection obviously guides and drives our work. Similarly, we propose that you proactively encounter this book rather than reactively respond to it.

You might pose to yourself questions raised in the following chapters. For instance: Do I fully recognize the hazards of my work? How often do I receive (or seek) nurturing relationships to offset the emotional toll of conducting therapy? Do I set realistic and appropriate boundaries for my work? For my private and family time? Have I considered and implemented the "healthy escapes" that my colleagues use and the research advocates? Beyond combating negative self-talk, how much cognitive restructuring do I use to keep myself on an even keel? What organizational changes have I made—or, more importantly, not made—to take care of myself? Should I return to personal therapy, participate in peer supervision, or seek more continuing education to keep myself vibrant professionally? And do I continue to stretch and grow as a psychotherapist? As a person?

Second on the list is the *intellectual predisposition* valued of the prospective psychotherapist (and psychotherapy book): rational thought, dispassionate examination, and disciplined objectivity. As authors, we have striven to disseminate factual, updated, and balanced information. As readers, you are urged to reexamine dispassionately your cherished beliefs (if not myths) in the light of scientific data. Half-truths and archaic stereotypes flourish in our discipline.

Families are not alone in shared myths; professions, consciously and unconsciously, collude in maintaining them. For example, many of us labor under the collective delusion that psychotherapists enter personal treatment, by and large, for training purposes and only during their graduate training. Rubbish! The majority of clinicians seek therapy once they are in practice and only rarely (about 10% of the time) for training (details in Chapter 10). For another example, many of us (especially men) suffer from the myth that easing the burdens of conducting psychotherapy is an individual and competitive task—to be handled alone, internally, like the solitary oak tree, without visible signs of distress. All our experience and the research, by contrast, point to the therapeutic value of interpersonal relationships, organizational changes, and collective action.

These and many other myths are partly the product of innocent ignorance, uninformed opinion. After all, how many of us took a graduate course on self-care? But these myths are also partly prejudice—willful ignorance—fanned by political considerations, gender stereotypes, paucity of reliable information, and inadequate discussion of caring for the person of the psychotherapist. We can do little here to pacify political and economic struggles, but we will try to present the topic with an intellectual predisposition.

Third and final on the Holt and Luborsky (1958) list is a *relativistic perspective*: the ability to accept individual differences, an appreciation for disparate contexts and values. You will find no uniformity myth (Kiesler, 1966; Norcross, 1988) of the therapist or treatment here. One size definitely does not fit all of us. A complex matrix of interacting variables—family background, training experiences, characterological vulnerabilities, sociodemographic diversity, professional discipline, personal values, practice setting, theoretical orientation, ad infinitum—reciprocally determine the eventual "distress" of the therapist. We present a large and integrated mixture of self-change methods throughout *Leaving It at the Office*, in recognition of the diverse needs and contexts of psychotherapists. The self-care strategies offered here represent a smorgasbord of sorts—a varied and tempting array of choices—but also more than that, since research has discovered that some strategies are more efficacious than others.

These, then, are three possible standards upon which to evaluate this undertaking (and prospective trainees): an introspective orientation, an intellectual predisposition, and a relativistic perspective.

A FEW WORDS ON STYLE

Those interested in the psychotherapist as a person have two principal sources of literature available to them, both representing incomplete extremes. The first is the periodic manuscript penned by practicing clinicians on their lives and experiences—autobiographical "kiss and tell" books, so to speak. The second is the formal research article presenting results of a group of responding therapists on a specific topic. The former typically suffers from egocentricity; the latter from statistical minutiae.

We have aimed for the middle ground to draw on the advantages of the polarities—the individual riches of the captivating life narrative and the nomothetic wisdom of the aggregate research. We thus interweave theoretical literature, survey data, empirical research, autobiographical material, and personal disclosures, including a few of our own. We have also recruited prominent therapists of diverse professions, genders, orientations, and ethnicities to share their stories on managing the inevitable hazards of conducting psychotherapy. The experiences and quotes of these "master therapists" are sprinkled liberally throughout the book.

These goals and our hybrid scientist-practitioner identity have led to a series of writing guidelines, as follows.

- *Form should parallel content.* The content of this book concerns the intimate and personal experiences of the psychotherapist; the writing, too, should be personal. A detached, objective view of the intimate, subjective life of the psychotherapist strikes us as incongruent.

- *Be data based.* This world of ours lacks many qualities, but notably these: data and humor. We value the insights of the great masters; however, we place empirical data and narrative truth above traditional authority. Colleagues discrediting replicated findings by branding them contrary to the observations of, say, Freud or Rogers or Beck do so at their own peril. Freud was certainly mistaken at times (and some would argue frequently), but it is not the duty of the pioneer to say the last word. Rather, the pioneer says the first word, and our task is to follow his line of inquiry faithfully by the host of clinical and research methods at our disposal (Guntrip, 1971).

- *Use humor on occasion.* If the profession of psychotherapy needs more solid data, then its practitioners need to laugh more. Psychotherapy has become a serious profession, perhaps too serious for our own good. As we discuss in Chapter 8, humor is one antidote for the stresses of the occupation and our occasional pomposity. Roald Dahl reminds us that "a little nonsense now and then is relished by the wisest men" (1972, p. 88). So accuse us of occasional jocularity, but we aspire to infuse data and humor into the subject and into the writing.

- *Focus on the content, not the researchers.* Traditional scholarship inadvertently highlights the surnames of researchers while subjugating

their findings. A psychiatric colleague once sarcastically characterized this as the "Smith (2005) sneezed, Jones (2006) burped, and in
reply, Smith (2007) farted" style of exposition. As much as possible,
we emphasize the content of our inquiry and relegate specific
names to the sidelines of parentheses.

- *Write in the present tense and with active verbs.* Much of our academic
  training has driven the unique, the emotional, and the active from
  our writing. As a consequence, professional writing has acquired
  a neutral, passive, and noncommittal flavor. Smith "reported,"
  "indicated," or "noted." Why not Smith "argues," "exclaims," or
  "writes"?

- *Minimize esoteric terms and ancient metaphors.* We have reduced the
  talismanic invocation of Greek myths and characters to six or seven
  occasions, and controlled the incessant word dropping, which
  sends our students scurrying to the dictionary for obscure etymol-
  ogy. But, as you probably just noticed, we do slip now and then and
  toss in a 50-cent term.

- *Write in the first person.* It is counterproductive to write on such a
  personal and intimate topic as self-care in the detached third person. We have decided to write in the first person plural—"we"—to
  convey the immediacy and individuality that the topic deserves.
  "We" is our convenient stand-in for one of us, both of us, and
  indeed, every one of us psychotherapists.

AT THE OFFICE, AWAY FROM THE OFFICE

Paradoxes abound when considering strategies to relieve the stress of conducting psychotherapy. Paradoxically, one way to *leave* distress at the
office is to enhance functioning *at* that same office—not to squeeze 10
hours of work frantically into 8 hours and then expect to retreat peace-
fully to a safe haven elsewhere, for instance. Paradoxically, too, one way to
leave distress *at* the office is to enhance one's life *outside* the office: enjoying your relationships, participating in healthy escapes, renewing your
spirituality, so that you are fully charged for the onslaught of intense contact with disturbed clients.

The upshot of these paradoxes is that a balanced and comprehensive
plan for your self-care as a mental health professional will require a dual
focus: in your workplace and outside your workplace. Accordingly, Chapters 2 through 12 are divided into sections labeled "at the office" and
"away from the office." Patients frequently act, for defensive purposes, as
though psychotherapists do not have lives outside the consulting room.
We shall not commit the same error.

INSTRUCTION MANUAL OR FIELD GUIDE?

Consistent with our relativistic perspective, we present more than one way to promote self-care. Life is not a uniform game with identical rules for all. Nor can problems be solved by mindlessly following a prescribed set of universal instructions. In *Zen and the Art of Motorcycle Maintenance*, Robert Pirsig (1974) put it this way:

> What's really angering about instructions of this sort is that they imply there's only one way to put this rotisserie together—their way. And that presumption wipes out all creativity. Actually there are hundreds of ways to put the rotisserie together and when they make you follow just one way without showing you the overall problem the instructions become hard to follow in such a way as not to make mistakes.

So it is, too, in alleviating the distress of conducting psychotherapy. We provide a broad and integrative scheme to enact self-care that can be—indeed must be—adapted to your individual needs and particular situation. In this sense, *Leaving It at the Office* is a field guide rather than an instruction manual.

As guides, we endeavor to cast light on the path ahead, chart the general geography, and warn of lurking dangers. Like the psychotherapists that we are and that you are (or are becoming), we offer interpersonal encouragement and specific guidance, but obviously cannot predict precisely what you will encounter. We can walk along with you, but cannot walk it for you—a sobering refrain of all clinicians. You will need to adapt this field guide, creatively and individually, to your unique journey.

The following 12 chapters summarize practitioner-recommended, field-tested, and research-informed methods of psychotherapist self-care. Unfortunately, the research on psychotherapist self-care has not progressed to the point where randomized clinical trials have been conducted. These chapters thus synthesize clinical wisdom, research literature, and therapist experience on self-care methods from disparate theoretical traditions. We also offer illustrative examples from our own practices and lives, as we struggle to practice what we preach (and research).

We hope that your spirit and practice will be touched as you read this book. These 12 self-care strategies, we hope, will reawaken and redirect sensitivities to the personal and professional identity of the psychotherapist. *Leaving It at the Office* can only exert its rightful purpose if you are embracing each moment with eager abandon! If our book has ignited your ability to do so, even by just a little bit, then our efforts will have been amply rewarded.

Acknowledgments

We are grateful to the many psychotherapists who, over the years, have participated in our research studies, attended our workshops, entered psychological treatment with us, and frequented our convention presentations. Their insights and experiences have shaped the recommendations found in this book. One cadre of master psychotherapists deserves special acknowledgment for participating in an intensive study on the ways they alleviate the distress of conducting psychotherapy:

Bernard D. Beitman, MD
Beth Brokaw, PhD
Russel Buskirk, MS
Nancy A. Caldwell, RN, MSW
Paul Clement, PhD
Rebecca C. Curtis, PhD
Albert Ellis, PhD
Barry A. Farber, PhD
Larry B. Feldman, MD
Herbert J. Freudenberger, PhD
Margaret Guy, MSW
Richard P. Halgin, PhD

Althea Horner, PhD
Florence W. Kaslow, PhD
Arnold A. Lazarus, PhD
Michael J. Mahoney, PhD
Alvin R. Mahrer, PhD
Kenneth Polite, PhD
Timothy Pylko, MD
Katherine S. Schnieder, PhD
Gary Schoener, MS
Margery Shelton, MSW
Diane Strausser, MSW
Neil Warren, PhD

Such research would be impossible without an army of capable collaborators and students. We wish to thank in this regard the members of our research teams for their multiple and essential contributions to this book. They include Joanie Laidig, Rene Cannon, Francis Healy, Rhonda Karg,

Paul Poelstra, Teri Stueland, Melissa Hedges, Maria Turkson, and Natalie Fala. A much larger number of psychotherapists—to this point 5,000 or 6,000 strong—were also indispensable members of our research team by sharing their experiences in our programmatic studies.

We were fortunate to recruit three of these stellar research assistants—now rising psychologists in their own right—to coauthor three of the chapters. Thank you, Drs. Rhonda Karg, Joan Laidig, and Maria Turkson.

We are indebted to hundreds of colleagues who have participated in our self-care workshops over the years. Three months following completion of each workshop, we e-mailed participants to "collegially prompt, encourage, and support your continued self-care as a psychotherapist. Hope this finds you engaging in more self-care—at least more than you did before the conference—and replenishing yourself from the slings and arrows of clinical work. If you have a minute and the inclination, I would enjoy hearing how, specifically, the workshop prompted you to think, act, or feel differently about your self-care." Their generous responses are sprinkled throughout the book. All responses, of course, are presented anonymously.

The editorial staff of The Guilford Press was of immeasurable assistance and infinite patience in bringing this volume to the light of published day. We extend our sincere gratitude, in particular, to Seymour Weingarten (Editor-in-Chief) and Jim Nageotte (Senior Editor). They have come to appreciate that the muses are not always on schedule.

Last but never least, we express our deepest appreciation to our life partners, Nancy and Joan, and to our children, Rebecca, Jonathon, Lisa, Julie, Jonathan, and William, to whom this book is dedicated. They have taught us the most fundamental and abiding lessons about balancing personal and professional lives. We are capable of *Leaving It at the Office* because of their caring and love.

Contents

CHAPTER 1

Valuing the Person of the Psychotherapist

Mental health professionals, by definition, study and modify human behavior. That is, we study and modify *other* humans. Psychological principles, methods, and research are rarely brought to bear on psychotherapists ourselves, with the probable exception of our unsolicited attempts to diagnose one another (Norcross, 2000).

Although understandable and explicable on many levels, this paucity of systematic study on psychotherapists' self-care is unsettling indeed. It is certainly less threatening, individually and collectively, to look outward rather than inward. Anna Freud once made the telling observation that becoming a psychotherapist was one of the most sophisticated defense mechanisms: granting us an aura of control and superiority and avoiding personal evaluation ourselves. In any case, this state of affairs strikes us as backwards: we should be studying ourselves and *then* others.

Consider that psychotherapists are among the most highly trained and experienced change agents. Yet, we know relatively little (at least publicly) about how we cope with our own distress or change our own behavior or struggle with the hazards of the craft. The tendency to view psychotherapists as not having lives outside the consulting room apparently afflicts us as well as our clients.

This book—and psychotherapist self-care—starts from the premise of *valuing the person of the psychotherapist*.

CONVERGENCE OF SCIENCE AND PRACTICE

The person of the psychotherapist is inextricably intertwined with treatment success. We know, scientifically and clinically, that the individual practitioner and the therapeutic relationship contribute to outcome at least as much as the particular treatment method. When not confounded with treatment, so-called therapist effects are large and frequently exceed treatment effects (Wampold, 2001, p. 200). Meta-analyses of therapist effects in psychotherapy outcome average 5–9% (Crits-Christoph et al., 1991; Wampold, 2001). A study estimated the variability of outcomes attributable to therapists in a managed care setting involving 6,146 patients and 581 therapists. About 5% of outcome was due to therapist effects; 0% was due to specific treatment (Wampold & Brown, 2005). Despite impressive attempts to experimentally render individual practitioners as controlled variables, it is simply not possible to mask the person and the contribution of the therapist.

That contribution of the individual therapist also entails the creation of a facilitative relationship with a patient. The therapeutic relationship, as every half-conscious practitioner knows in her bones, is the indispensable soil of the treatment enterprise. Best statistical estimates are that the therapeutic relationship, including empathy, collaboration, the alliance, and so on, accounts for approximately 10% of psychotherapy outcome (Norcross, 2002). That rivals or exceeds the proportion of outcome attributable to the particular treatment method.

Suppose we asked a neutral scientific panel from outside the field to review the corpus of psychotherapy research to determine what is the most powerful phenomenon we should be studying, practicing, and teaching. That panel (Henry, 1998, p. 128)

> would find the answer obvious, and *empirically validated*. As a general trend across studies, the largest chunk of outcome variance not attributable to pre-existing patient characteristics involves individual therapist differences and the emergent therapeutic relationship between patient and therapist, regardless of technique or school of therapy. This is the main thrust of three decades of empirical research.

Here is a quick clinical exemplar to drive the point home. It derives from a thought experiment we use in our clinical workshops. We ask participants, "What accounts for the success of psychotherapy?" And then we ask, "What accounts for the success of your personal therapy?" The prototypical answer is "Many things account for success, including the patient, the therapist, their relationship, the treatment method, and the context." But when pressed, approximately 90% will answer "the relationship."

Their responses dovetail perfectly with the hundreds of published studies that have asked clients to describe what was helpful in their psychotherapy. Patients routinely identify the therapeutic relationship. Clients do not emphasize the effectiveness of particular techniques or methods; instead, they primarily attribute the effectiveness of their treatment to the relationship with their therapists (Elliott & James, 1989).

Consider the clients' perspectives on the helpful aspects of their treatment in the classic National Institute of Mental Health (NIMH) Collaborative Treatment Study of Depression. Even among patients receiving manualized treatments in a large research study, the most common responses fell into the categories of "My therapist helped" (41%) and "I learned something new" (36%). At posttreatment, fully 32% of the patients receiving placebo plus clinical management wrote that the most helpful part of their "treatment" was their therapists (Gershefski, Arnkoff, Glass, & Elkin, 1996).

As a final illustration, we would point to studies on the most informed consumers of psychotherapy—psychotherapists themselves. In two of our studies in the United States and Great Britain, hundreds of psychotherapists reflected on their own psychotherapy experiences and nominated lasting lessons they acquired concerning the practice of psychotherapy (Norcross, Strausser-Kirtland, & Missar, 1988; Norcross, Drydan, & DeMichele, 1992). The most frequent responses all concerned the interpersonal relationships and dynamics of psychotherapy: the centrality of warmth, empathy, and the personal relationship; the importance of transference and countertransference; the inevitable humanness of the therapist; and the need for more patience in psychotherapy. Conversely, a review of published studies that identified covariates of harmful therapies received by mental health professionals concluded that the harm was typically attributed to distant and rigid therapists, emotionally seductive therapists, and poor patient–therapist matches (Orlinsky, Norcross, Rønnestad, & Wiseman, 2005).

All of this is to say that science and practice impressively converge on the conclusion that the person of the clinician is the locus of successful psychotherapy. It is neither grandiosity nor self-preoccupation that leads us to psychotherapist self-care; it is the incontrovertible science and practice that demands we pursue self-care.

Want to improve the effectiveness of psychotherapy? Then follow the evidence, the evidence that insists we select, train, and nourish the individual practitioner.

CONFLUENCE OF INDIVIDUAL AND ENVIRONMENT

A leitmotif of this book is the interdependence of the person and the environment in determining effective self-care. The self-care and burnout fields have been polarized into rival camps. One camp focuses on the individual's deficits—the "fault, dear Brutus, is in ourselves" advocates—and correspondingly recommends individualistic solutions to self-care; a second camp focuses on the systemic and organizational pressures—the "impossible profession with inhumane demands" advocates—and naturally recommends environmental and social solutions. In this book, we value both camps and adopt an interactional perspective that recognizes the reciprocal confluence of person-in-the-environment. The self is always in a system.

When conceptualizing the self-in-a-system, we repeatedly point to the unique motives, family of origins, and underlying psychodynamics of mental health professionals. What drives a person to concern him- or herself with the dark side of the human psyche? What is it that compels certain people to elect to help those who are suffering, wounded, or dysfunctional? Assuredly they are a "special sort," since the average person prefers to downplay the psychic sufferings of fellow humans and avoid extensive contact with troubled individuals (Norcross & Guy, 1989).

The question of motivation—why did I (really) become a psychotherapist?—is obviously not a simple or entirely conscious one. To be sure, the altruistic motive "to help people" is one cornerstone of the vocational choice, but it is incomplete. It begs the deeper questions: Why is "helping people" of utmost concern for you? What makes it a deeply satisfying experience? Of all the helping careers—assisting the homeless, saving the environment, rendering public service, teaching the uneducated, tending to physical ills—why *this* career as a psychotherapist? Even the most saintly among us is moved by a complex stew of motives, some admirable and some less so, some conscious and some less so. Psychotherapists frequently report that they come to realize the reasons they chose their discipline only well into their careers or during the course of intensive personal therapy (Holt & Luborsky, 1958).

The failure to consider the individual motives, needs, and vulnerabilities of psychotherapists renders much of the well-intended practical advice on self-care hollow and general. To paraphrase Freud, it's akin to giving a starving person a dinner menu. One-size-fits-all treatments never accommodate many people, be it our clients or ourselves. In *Leaving It at the Office*, we strive to present self-care in the context of, and responsive to, the emotional vulnerabilities and resources of the individual clinician.

RUNNING AGAINST THE TIDE

Even as we write this chapter, we are painfully aware that our message runs counter to the zeitgeist of the industrialization of mental health care. Managed care devalues the individuality of the practitioner, preferring instead to speak of "providers" on "panels." The pervasive medical model prefers manualized treatments for DSM diagnoses to therapeutic relationships with unique humans. The evidence-based practice movement highlights the evidence in favor of specific treatments and downplays the evidence for the curative powers of the human clinician (and patient). Our emphasis on valuing the person of the therapist may seem a nostalgic throwback to the 1970s and 1980s.

At the same time, we detect a dawning recognition, really a reawakening, that the therapist herself is the focal process of change. "The inescapable fact of the matter is that the therapist is a person, however much he may strive to make himself an instrument of his patient's treatment" (Orlinsky & Howard, 1977, p. 567). This book stands firmly against the encroaching tide of the tyranny of technique and the myth of disembodied treatment.

The pursuit of technical competency has much to recommend it, but it may inadvertently subordinate the value of the personal formation and maturation of the psychologist (Norcross, 2005b). The ongoing march toward evidence-based practices tends to neglect the human dimension of the practitioner and the psychotherapy. It has created an environment where, as Thoreau complains in *Walden* (1854, p. 25), "men have become the tools of their tools." Movements that address only, or primarily, the techniques of psychotherapy quickly become arid, disembodied, and technical enterprises.

Lest we be misunderstood on this point, let us reveal our bias, a bias rooted in years of conducting psychotherapy and research. Effective practice in mental health will embrace the treatment method, the individual therapist, the therapy relationship, the patient, and their optimal combinations (Norcross & Lambert, 2005). We value the power of the individual therapist, but not only that. As integrative psychotherapists, we try to avoid the ubiquitous pull toward dichotomous and polarizing characterizations of the evidence. The evidence tells us that successful psychotherapy is a product of many components, all of which revolve around, and depend upon, the individual psychotherapist. That's good science *and* good relationships.

SELF-CARE AS ETHICAL IMPERATIVE

For those not convinced or only partially convinced by the scientific evidence on the person of the psychotherapist, we now turn to self-care's ethical imperative. Every ethical code of mental health professionals includes a provision or two about the need for self-care. The American Psychological Association's Ethical Code (2002), for example, directs psychologists to maintain an awareness "of the possible effect of their own physical and mental health on their ability to help those with whom they work" (p. 1062). One section (2.06) of the code instructs psychologists, when they become aware of personal problems that may interfere with performing work-related duties adequately, to "take appropriate measures, such as obtaining professional consultation or assistance, and determine whether they should limit, suspend, or terminate their work-related duties" (p. 1064).

The American Counseling Association's (2005) Code of Ethics, for another example, enjoins counselors to "engage in self-care activities to maintain and promote their emotional, physical, mental, and spiritual well-being to best meet their professional responsibilities" (p. 9). Further, the code states, "Counselors are alert to the signs of impairment from their own physical, mental, or emotional problems and refrain from offering or providing professional services when such impairment is likely to harm a client or others. They seek assistance for problems that reach the level of professional impairment . . . " (p. 9).

Without attending to our own care, we will not be able to help others and prevent harm to them. Psychotherapist self-care is a critical prerequisite for patient care. In other words, self-care is not simply a personal matter but also an ethical necessity, a moral imperative (Barnett, Johnston, & Hillard, 2006; Carroll, Gilroy, & Murra, 1999). We gently urge you to challenge the morality of self-sacrifice at all costs and to consider the indispensability of self-care.

THE PARADOXES OF SELF-CARE

> Suppose you were to come upon a man in the woods working feverishly to saw down a tree. "What are you doing?" you ask. "Can't you see?" comes the impatient reply. "I'm sawing down this tree." You exclaim: "You look exhausted! How long have you been at it?" The man replies: "Over 5 hours, and I'm beat! This is hard work." You inquire: "Well, why don't you take a break for a few minutes and sharpen that saw? I'm sure it would go a lot faster." The man emphatically replies: "I don't have time to sharpen the saw. I'm too busy sawing!"

That is the first paradox of self-care: no time to sharpen the saw! The story, incidentally, comes from Stephen Covey's (1989, p. 287) *The 7 Habits of Highly Effective People*. It is *sooo* easy to see and diagnose it in other people; it is *sooo* hard to get off the treadmill ourselves.

Existential–humanistic psychotherapists Sapienza and Bugental (2000, p. 459) put the self-care paradox bluntly: "Many of us have never really learned how to take the time to care and to nourish ourselves, having been trained to believe that this would be selfish. . . . Nor have most psychologists taken the time to develop compassion for themselves, and compassion for their wounds."

Not that psychotherapists are opposed to self-care; far from it. Instead, we are busy, multitasking professionals dedicated to helping others but who frequently cannot locate the time to help ourselves. Clients, families, paperwork, colleagues, students, and friends seem to always assume priority. The ideal balance of caring for others *and* for ourselves tends to favor the former. At the risk of redundancy, we believe it begins with prioritizing the value of yourself as a person/psychotherapist.

The point segues into another paradox of psychotherapist self-care: Not availing ourselves of what we provide or recommend to clients. We oftimes feel hypocritical or duplicitous—suggesting to others that they work less, exercise more, renew themselves, and so forth—while we do not take our own advice. How often do we sit with patients, encouraging them to "relax and take a vacation," while calculating in our own case our lost therapy revenue and airfare and concluding that we can't afford to take the time away from the office right now (Penzer, 1984)?

A representative example from one of our workshop participants is instructive:

"I had the ergonomic person here yesterday for an analysis in my office, thanks to back pain that signaled something negative to me. When I had to answer her questions about my amount of work, vacation, and so on, it was embarrassing! How could I possibly with a good conscience give a talk on stress management when I behave as I do?"

On a positive note, the person optimistically concluded that "I'm assuming the universe is sending me needed messages and that your reminder e-mail about self-care is yet another."

A recurrent theme of our book is the acknowledgment that it is easier to be wise and mature for others than for ourselves. If you are still feeling a little hypocritical, sheepish, or guilty about not practicing what you preach, then join us and the crowd. We are far more adept at recommending self-care to others than practicing it ourselves, as our families and friends will readily attest. Until quite lately in our own lives, self-care was regrettably more of a research proficiency than a personal accomplishment. We are in no position to moralize.

In fact, we take seriously an early lesson of folks traveling to Esalen, the human potential center in California. Although the trainers at Esalen were teaching people how to relate to themselves and other people in optimal ways, they themselves had serious difficulties in their own lives and relationships. This led Richard Price to popularize what he called Esalen's Law: we always teach others what we most need to learn ourselves. A corollary is that each of us is our own worst student. (Thanks to Ken Pope for reminding us of the law's origins.)

Psychotherapists frequently comment on the cruel irony of giving to clients precisely what they deprive their families of. One therapist (Penzer, 1984, p. 54) notes the dissonance inherent in "spending several hours a day playing Uno, Checkers, and War in the name of play therapy and coming home in the evening and casting my children's requests aside in the name of fatigue." Another colleague was conducting psychotherapy with a harried middle-aged father one evening and focusing on the father's need to spend more time with his son and daughter. Alas, the therapist was seeing patients four evenings a week and ignoring his own young children! Many therapists will candidly admit to giving more time, energy, and devotion to their practices than to their spouses, children, or themselves (Penzer, 1984). Clearly, the lesson is one of "Physician, take thine own medicine."

Just as being a lawyer does not necessarily make one more honest and being a physician does not necessarily make one healthier (Goldberg, 1992), so too being a psychotherapist does *not* make one automatically more proficient at self-care. In fact, it is frequently the converse in a profession in which people enter "to help others."

RESEARCH ON PSYCHOTHERAPIST SELF-CARE

We have been researching the self-care and self-change of mental health professionals for the past 25 years. These studies have occupied sizable portions of our professional careers and, not coincidentally, our personal lives. We and our colleagues have conducted numerous studies to identify what distinguishes the self-change of mental health professionals from that of educated laypersons, to survey practitioners about what they use and don't use to soothe themselves, to discern what change principles are particularly effective for therapist self-care, and to interview seasoned psychotherapists about their personal struggles and salvations. We have taken the Socratic dicta of "know thyself" and "heal thyself" to heart—and to the lab. The resultant compilation of self-care strategies is clinician-recommended, research-informed, and practitioner-tested.

Some of our earliest research, including one of our doctoral dissertations (Norcross & Prochaska, 1986a, 1986b), was premised, mostly unconsciously, on the fantasy that psychotherapists' clinical skills would inoculate us from the inevitable stressors of living. But all of the research results have regrettably disabused us of this fantasy. Psychotherapists experience the same frequency of life disruptions as educationally and economically comparable laypersons. We also furtively hoped that our research would compellingly demonstrate that psychotherapists were better self-changers than mere mortals. But here, too, we were ruefully disappointed: this is simply not the case. In truth, we psychotherapists cope just a tad more effectively with life disruptions than laypersons with similar education, which comes as an insult to our narcissism, no doubt!

A therapist-patient of ours employed at a health maintenance organization was treating 33 patients a week at the HMO, seeing patients three nights a week in private practice, and teaching a course on another night. He then complained of feeling exhausted and overwhelmed. Duh! His complaints followed a psychotherapy session in which another of our patients, a very hard-working teacher, stayed up past midnight creating her own Christmas bows and then complaining of exhaustion. We are not so different from our patients—we are all more human than otherwise.

A question that persistently arises and that many of you may be silently asking is "But what about our theoretical orientations? Won't our preferred systems of psychotherapy affect how we care for ourselves?" We have conducted multiple studies on this topic during the past 25 years (see Norcross & Aboyoun, 1994, for a review). The results will probably surprise you, as they certainly did us.

In treating patients, psychotherapists use change principles in accordance with their theoretical orientation. Cognitive-behavioral therapists, for example, report using counterconditioning, contingency management, and stimulus control significantly more than colleagues of eclectic, psychodynamic, and humanistic persuasions. On the other hand, psychodynamic therapists rely more on the therapy relationship and catharsis than do their behavioral colleagues. That the treatment of clients varies predictably with orientation is not surprising and, in fact, is quite expected.

The question then arose: Are psychotherapists equally influenced by theories in treating themselves, in their own self-care? Apparently not. We have been unable to discern any significant orientation differences in psychotherapists' self-care. This pattern of results has now been replicated in five separate studies involving different disorders and professions. Indeed, we have been unable to discern even a few statistically significant differences expected by chance alone. In toto, these composite findings strongly argue for a considerable similarity among psychotherapists in their own self-care, independent of their theories.

We can offer three interpretations for this pattern of findings (Norcross, Prochaska, & Hambrecht, 1991). The first interpretation comes from attribution research. Just as there are stable disparities in attributions for people in the roles of actors and observers, so too there appear to be robust differences in change strategies for people in the roles of clinicians and clients. In their role as psychotherapists, people rely heavily on theories for facilitating change in others. In their role as self-changers, people are not as influenced by theoretical prescriptions.

A second interpretation reflects a cynical perspective on the disparities between psychotherapists' public careers and their personal lives. That is, psychotherapists may not avail themselves of what they offer their patients. Theoretical orientations may be for treatment-facilitated change of clients, not for self-initiated change of themselves. Negatively stated, one may *not* necessarily have to "practice what one preaches." As George Kelly (1955) noted many years ago, psychotherapists do *not* apply their theories reflexively. That is, they do not apply the same theories to their own behavior as psychotherapists that they use in understanding and treating patients.

The third and more positive explanation is that psychotherapists become more pragmatic, eclectic, and "secular" when they confront their own distress. This view is reminiscent of early psychotherapy process research that suggested experienced psychotherapists behave and think quite similarly (e.g., Fiedler, 1950a, 1950b) and also reminiscent of a "therapeutic underground" (Wachtel, 1977), an unofficial consensus of what experienced clinicians believe to be true. Psychotherapists may well value clinical strategies quite different from what they offer their clients or from what they consider to be within their professional competence. On a personal level, clinicians may be taking psychotherapy integration to heart (Norcross & Goldfried, 2005).

George Stricker (1995), a friend and a prominent psychodynamicist, has written movingly about just such a personal integration in self-care. George and several fellow psychotherapists rented a small, puddle-jumping airplane in South America for an intimate view of the spectacular Iguazu waterfalls. George began experiencing some panic symptoms as he looked over the falls to appreciate the beauty that led them there in the first place. He realized his training and proficiency in psychodynamic therapy were not particularly useful for self-management of acute panic. Ever the pragmatic integrationist, George immediately became a cognitive-behavioral therapist with the assistance of his colleagues and successfully ameliorated his anxiety. He still employs some of the cognitive-behavioral methods he was taught, when faced with similar situations. Not a cure, to be sure, but a good way of dealing with situational anxieties.

Also consistent with this pragmatic and integrative explanation is the repeated finding that many psychotherapists choose a type of personal therapy different from what they practice themselves (see Chapter 10, and Norcross & Grunebaum, 2005). The majority of behavior therapists, in particular, choose *non*behavioral personal therapy. Practitioners, it appears, have learned that rival orientations are complimentary, not contradictory, when it comes to their own health.

Our decades of research on self-care also lead us to emphasize self-care principles or strategies, as opposed to techniques. One of the lessons from our research is that effective psychotherapist self-care is characterized by a complex, differential pattern of strategies. These strategies or principles represent an intermediate level of abstraction between concrete techniques and global theory. There are literally thousands of self-care techniques (e.g., meditation, assertion, dream analysis, vacations), and, Lord knows, we cannot agree on a single theory (e.g., psychoanalysis, cognitive, systemic, narrative); however, research increasingly reveals that we can agree on broad principles. Given the diversity of individual preferences and available resources, we recommend broad strategies as opposed to specific techniques.

If a colleague is plagued by occupational anxieties, the research suggests that the strategies of healthy escapes and helping relationships may well prove effective. Once the strategies are identified, then the individual practitioner can discover for herself the available and preferred techniques for implementing these strategies—for instance, massage, exercise, and meditation for healthy alternatives and peer support groups or clinical supervision for helping relationships. The focus should be squarely placed on broad strategies, which you then adapt to your own situation and preferences (Norcross, 2000).

Our research has additionally shown appreciable outcome differences among various psychotherapist self-care strategies, but the effect of any *single* strategy is rather modest. The different change strategies that people bring to bear on their distress do make a difference. The 12 self-care strategies recommended in this book are demonstrably more effective than the passive strategies of, say, wishful thinking, self-blame, and substance abuse (Norcross & Aboyoun, 1994). At the same time, there is no single self-care strategy so outstandingly effective that its possession alone would ensure an ability to conquer distress. These findings suggest to us, as they have to others, that possessing a particular skill in one's arsenal is less important than having a variety of self-care strategies. Seasoned practitioners have extended valuable lessons from their clinical work to their personal lives: avoid concentration on a single theory and promote cognitive and experiential growth on a broad front.

The overarching moral to be derived from our research is that psychotherapists should avail themselves of multiple self-care strategies unencumbered by theoretical dictates. Take psychotherapy integration to heart; that is, embrace multiple strategies associated with diverse theoretical traditions. Be comprehensive, flexible, and secular in replenishing yourself. The self-care strategies compiled in *Leaving It at the Office* are theoretically neutral and blend psychotherapists' in-the-trenches recommendations with the nascent empirical findings.

BEGIN WITH SELF-AWARENESS
AND SELF-MONITORING

Quantitative studies and interview surveys alike confirm the conventional wisdom on the centrality of self-monitoring our own distress and, concomitantly, our own self-care. In one illustrative study, both program directors and professional psychologists identified "self-awareness/self-monitoring" as the top-ranked contributor to their optimal functioning (Schwebel & Coster, 1998). In another study of master therapists, self-awareness was deeply embedded in, and routinely prized as a prerequisite for, professional conduct (Skovholt & Jennings, 2004).

Becoming aware, as we usefully remind our patients, is the key first step. In a monumental multinational study of psychotherapist development over the lifespan (Orlinsky & Rønnestad, 2005, p. 200), the authors pointedly conclude:

> As a final recommendation, then, we restate how important it is that practitioners of all professions and theoretical orientations *consistently monitor and carefully attend to their sense of current professional development and their level of satisfaction with therapeutic work.* (italics in original)

Assess your own self-care as you might a student's or a patient's self-care. Be prepared to be shocked by the results. You spend most of your day in intimate contact with distressed patients, anxious parents, and insensitive administrators? You work *how* many hours per week?! Your last non-convention vacation was when?! You never get lunch at the office?! And then you take work home with you and receive calls at night?!

Structured questionnaires can serve as convenient, empirically grounded measures in facilitating systematic self-reflection (Orlinsky & Rønnestad, 2005). Practitioners might use questionnaires to monitor their own work morale and establish benchmarks for detecting signs of stagnation or decline. Student therapists might use them privately to monitor their own clinical functioning and development and share the results with supervisors. Supervisors, in turn, might use them in parallel fashion to track supervisee's distress, self-care, and development. (See Appendix E in Orlinsky & Rønnestad, 2005, for sample questionnaires, scoring keys, and norms for psychotherapists; or consider one of the burnout instruments, such as the Maslach Burnout Inventory.)

Many practitioners find it useful to track their self-care through writing, journaling, or logging (e.g., Baker, 2003; Williams-Nickelson, 2006). Some prefer structured self-monitoring on a specific behavior, such as food diaries, mood and self-talk logs, or exercise calendars. Others prefer a narrative journal of feelings and experiences. Meta-analyses on the effects of expressive writing find (small) positive effects on physical and psychological outcomes (e.g., Frisina, Borod, & Lepore, 2004; Sloan & Marx, 2004). In any case, a written chronicle improves adherence to a self-care regimen (DiMatteo, 2006)—of course, so long as maintaining the journal or log does not itself become yet another onerous responsibility or compulsive pursuit.

Gerald (Jerry) Corey, author of several influential textbooks on counseling, exemplifies the self-monitoring of work and play. For years, Jerry has recorded the time devoted to work and to exercise (walking and biking). Since the year 2000, he has averaged 41 hours of work weekly and an impressive 12.6 hours of exercise weekly. Jerry testifies that logging his work and exercise time keeps him more honest, balanced, and motivated.

Self-awareness can be augmented by contracting for some honest feedback from loved ones about our work week. Self-awareness does not imply that we go it alone, only that we must become aware and own our behavior. For some of us, self-monitoring entails attending (nondefensively, if possible) to interpersonal feedback from significant others about our functioning. In our case, we attend to our spouses' observations that we are looking haggard, working longer hours, or traveling too often to supplement our own monitoring. In the early years, our defenses were immediately activated, and we quickly rationalized with such feeble protests as "Well, I have a responsible position!", "But it's not as bad as Jim's schedule," and the ever handy "Next week will be easier."

Awareness alone, however, is not sufficient. Self-care readily becomes one of those "healthy oughts," like flossing teeth and getting sleep, that gets discussed and then discarded. Here's how one workshop participant characterized his history of neglecting self-care:

> "Somehow my wonderful plans and desires based on my emotions did not materialize. I yet once more realize the various steps in actual life transformation. Awareness is not enough, and understanding is only the beginning of the essential first step."

In several of our studies devoted to discovering the successful self-change strategies of psychotherapists, self-liberation—a fancy name for choosing and self-realization—consistently emerged as an effective strategy. This strategy entails the choice of changing and the ensuing responsibility. It is the acknowledgment, the commitment, and the burden of replenishing yourself, professionally and personally.

In the prophetic words of a participant in one of our self-care workshops: "Your presentation was a necessary reminder to me that I cannot just advocate attention to self-care for my staff or assume that it will stay in my consciousness without some intention. I need to apply it, more consciously and intentionally, to myself. It caused me to reconsider things I was and was not doing to engage in self-care." That, in a nutshell, is precisely our intention.

To reach the action stage of sustained behavior change (Prochaska, Norcross, & DiClemente, 1995), awareness and self-monitoring must beget a proactive choice. Good intentions must concretely translate into healthy behaviors. "I find that it really works to write in my exercise time on my calendar each day and make that a really important time," as one colleague told us. In other words, we must make self-care a priority.

MAKING SELF-CARE A PRIORITY

It begins with reminding busy practitioners of the personal and professional need to tend to their own psychological health. Call it valuing, prizing, prioritizing, or another action verb, but find a way of building it into the mainstream of your life. Self-care is not a narcissistic luxury to be fulfilled as time permits; it is a human requisite, a clinical necessity, and an ethical imperative.

If not us, then who will value our self-care? Certainly not our clients, who neurotically would bleed us to death if permitted. Certainly not insurance carriers, who greedily demand more of us while doling out less reimbursement and less autonomy. Hopefully our loved ones, but they understandably have their own needs and agendas, which only partially match ours. No, if anyone is to advocate for and prioritize self-care, it must be us.

Self-awareness and self-monitoring should beget self-empathy: the capacity to notice, value, and respond to our own needs as generously as we attend to the needs of others (Murphy & Dillon, 2002). Many practitioners blame themselves for feeling drained and then, to complicate the drain, berate themselves for feeling that way. Please develop self-empathy, taking the time and space for yourself without feeling selfish, guilty, or needy.

Consider the daily life of the "successful" busy psychotherapist in independent practice. Up early and tending to family matters. Off in a rush to the office to "catch up," return telephone calls, and complete insurance forms. Confronting an avalanche of suffering patients and juggling them with the emergencies. Squeezing in a part-time teaching, supervision, or consultation commitment. Working several evenings, perhaps even a weekend day. Taking calls at nights, completing paperwork at home.

Or consider the committed "successful" clinician working at a community mental health center. One of our workshop participants characterized her agency as one "that would chew me up and spit me out, then ask that I reassemble myself so they could have dessert. It is impossible to do what I am asked to do. I am salaried and work far more than 40 hours a week (from 45 to 50 hours)."

Or the pastoral counselor who wrote us recently about his new position at a hospital as

> "a chaplain, and it is mega stressful. I am on call for 104 hours per week. There are people dying of cancer and other diseases every day. This week I have been working with a young couple when doctors turned the life-support machine off on their little baby. The baby was supposed to die (they had all said their good-byes), but it surprisingly lived. So, the young couple were left not knowing whether to feel sad or glad since the baby had significant irreversible brain damage.

After dealing with that situation, I felt terrible, and I am not sure what could help me afterward, let alone the couple."

All are working overscheduled lives. Skimping on breakfast, probably skipping lunch, existing on snack foods during the day on the run. Running nearly on empty, subclinically exhausted. Little time for self or loved ones. In a success-driven culture hostile to rest and self-care, many psychotherapists have lost the balance, priorities, and mission they once treasured. *Quis custodiet ipsos custodies?* (Who will guard the guards?)

A simple and surprisingly effective method for prioritizing self-care is to make the calendar work for you. Schedule the activities that matter most to you on your calendar (Weiss, 2004). One of our master therapists told us that "I write down the consequential before the mundane in my schedule book. My lunches with friends, exercise times, and family events are there every month." Of course, putting something *into* your schedule typically means taking something *out* of your schedule. That active choice entails both pain and freedom.

The goal is not simply to survive but to thrive in practice and as a psychotherapist (Pope & Vasquez, 2005). Not only to keep your nose above the waterline, but to swim naturally and joyfully.

Our goal leads us, curiously enough, to barely mention how to "avoid burnout" in this book. That would be equivalent to discussing how to avoid catching a cold, how to avoid a bad marriage, or how to avoid an automobile accident. Trying to avoid burnout, while noble in intent, is avoidant as a strategy, reflective of a psychopathology orientation, and negative in orientation. As one of our workshop participants wrote, "It was important to hear you refocus self-care away from the negative of avoiding burnout toward actually living well." Exactly so.

Our message is that it is far more productive to promote self-care. Sure, we can temporarily alleviate the distress of clinical work; but, more optimistically and proactively, we can value and grow the person of the psychotherapist.

SELF-CARE CHECKLIST

✓ Adhere to the ethical imperative of engaging in "self-care activities to maintain and promote your emotional, physical, mental, and spiritual well-being to best meet your professional responsibilities" (American Counseling Association, 2005, p. 9).

✓ Ask your patients, if you have not done so recently, what has been most helpful in their psychotherapy. Take to heart their frequent compliments about your presence, affirmation, and support.

✓ Resist the pressures of managed care to define yourself as a nameless and disembodied "provider" of mental health services. Maintain your individual identity as a distinctive practitioner of psychological healing.

✓ Internalize the relational crux of the work. Yes, we conduct treatments to eradicate DSM disorders, but we also offer relationships that heal people.

✓ Assess your deep motives for becoming a psychotherapist beyond the altruism of "to help people." How are these motives facilitating or hindering your effective self-care?

✓ Prioritize your self-care: put specific times in your schedule to sharpen the saw.

✓ Develop self-empathy: the capacity to notice, value, and respond to your own needs as generously as you attend to the needs of clients.

✓ Practice what you preach to your clients about nourishing the self: avail yourself (when applicable) of what you provide or recommend to clients with similar needs.

✓ Embrace an integrative mix of effective self-care strategies (as opposed to relying on a single theoretical orientation).

✓ Avoid concentrating on a single self-care technique, and promote cognitive and experiential growth on a broad front. Do you rely on only one or two self-care methods?

✓ Assess your own self-care as you might a student's or a patient's self-care—on a weekly or monthly basis.

✓ Track your self-care by maintaining a journal, calendar, or behavioral log of activity.

✓ Complete structured questionnaires on burnout and self-care periodically to facilitate your self-awareness and self-monitoring.

✓ Contract for some honest feedback from significant others about your work week, functioning, and self-care. Let others supplement and enhance your self-monitoring.

✓ Put your consequential self-care activities in your schedule/calendar first thing every month. Literally schedule your self-care.

✓ Alleviate the distress of conducting psychotherapy, to be sure, but also value and grow the person of the psychotherapist.

RECOMMENDED READING

Farber, B. A., & Norcross, J. C. (Eds.). (2005). Why I (really) became a psychotherapist. *Journal of Clinical Psychology: In Session, 61*(8).

Guy, J. D. (1987). *The personal life of the psychotherapist.* New York: Wiley.

Norcross, J. C., & Aboyoun, D. C. (1994). Self-change experiences of psychothera-pists. In T. M. Brinthaupt & R. P. Lipka (Eds.), *Changing the self.* Albany: State University of New York Press.

Pope, K. S., & Vasquez, M. J. T. (2005). *How to survive and thrive as a therapist: Information, ideas, and resources for psychologists in practice.* Washington, DC: American Psychological Association.

The therapist as a person. On Dr. Ken Pope's website at *kspope.com/therapistas/index.php.*

CHAPTER 2

Refocusing on the Rewards

"Sometimes I wonder . . . why did I decide to become a psychothera-pist? Has it satisfied my expectations? For the most part I must say 'yes.' Of course, there have been moments of discouragement and disappointment. At times I've even thought about selling real estate or becoming a financial planner instead! But most of the time, I'm very happy to be a psychotherapist. In fact, I don't know of any other career that would suit me as well."

So said one of our master clinicians in our interviews. She speaks for most of us in saying that psychotherapy is a very satisfying and rewarding career.

Clients are not the only ones changed by psychotherapy. We practi-tioners feel enriched, nourished, and privileged in conducting psycho-therapy. The work brings relief, joy, meaning, growth, vitality, and genu-ine engagement, both for our patients and for ourselves.

Pause for a moment to think back to the emotional and vocational process that led you to decide to become a psychotherapist. For some, this occurred at an early age out of a desire to help those in distress. For oth-ers, there was a gradual evolution toward this particular helping role. It was likely motivated by a number of factors that included a realization of the considerable rewards and satisfactions associated with clinical work.

For most mental health professionals, there continues to be a strong sense of purpose in their ongoing commitment to the role of psychotherapist. Although the reasons for remaining in practice and the sources of satisfaction may change over the years, the underlying sense of purpose and meaning usually remains the same.

As a group, psychotherapists are quite satisfied with their career choice (Guy, 1987). Cross-sectional and longitudinal research of career satisfaction among psychotherapists reveals consistent and high levels of satisfaction (Walfish, Moritz, & Stenmark, 1991). In one of our studies of clinical psychologists (Norcross, Karpiak, & Santoro, 2005), the percentage of those who expressed satisfaction was no lower than 88% at any time over the past 44 years. That number compares quite favorably to physicians who provide direct patient care (Landon, Reschovsky, & Blumenthal, 2003). In that study, 80% of primary care physicians and 81% of specialists reported some level of satisfaction. Put simply, most psychotherapists are satisfied with their careers and would enter the same field if they had to choose all over again.

Lasting satisfaction is associated with clinical work, particularly after the practitioner has been in practice for more than 10 years. Perhaps this satisfaction reflects a growing sense of confidence that overcomes the feeling of being a charlatan or an imposter, a phenomenon frequently reported by neophytes. Experienced psychotherapists have probably also learned how to avoid or lessen the impact of the hazards we outline in the next chapter. Regardless of the reasons, once the psychotherapist has passed the 10-year mark, he or she has probably achieved a degree of satisfaction and success that is likely to continue throughout the remainder of her career.

Many of the factors that originally led to the decision to enter the profession also keep the clinician committed to continuing in this career. The majority of our master psychotherapists indicated in our interviews that refocusing on the rewards of practicing psychotherapy enabled them to reduce their work-related distress. These positive aspects of clinical practice revitalize the practitioner's spirit and renew her commitment, particularly after the novelty of the work has worn off. As one master clinician put it: "I have a great love for what I do. When the job gets stressful, for whatever reason, I focus on how much I love my work. That helps me reduce my stress and continue."

Another of our master therapists expressed the identical sentiment in more detail:

> "There are times when things are not going well with a particular patient, and I may feel ignorant, nonhelpful, frustrated, or even like a bit of a sham. I need to remind myself of a couple of things, like that I have helped a number of individuals. I need to remind myself about

the intimacy of the work, the wonderful opportunity to help others, the rewards of the work. These include helpful intimacy. Therapy is one of those few professions where one can get paid for doing something that feels good. It feels productive and meaningful. If I am stuck, I'll either think of work I've done with others or work that I have done with this particular person that in the past has gotten us to a point where we feel more connected than we are at the moment."

When looking for ways to alleviate the distress of practicing psychotherapy, it is useful to begin by recalling your reasons for entering the profession in the first place. Much like reminding yourself of why you fell in love with your partner, such reflection on your role as a psychotherapist can refresh your sense of calling.

Similarly, when planning and practicing self-care, it is essential to recall the multiple rewards of practice. However, humans tend to react more strongly to—and probably have a longer memory for—aversive events (Kramen-Kahn & Hansen, 1998); so, we must highlight the overlooked rewards and facilitate recall of the successes. Following our review of the rewards of practicing psychotherapy, we offer several specific methods of recalling our original mission and of refocusing on the rewards of our craft.

REWARDS AT THE OFFICE

The typical workday for some psychotherapists is widely varied, including an array of tasks and challenges that take the practitioner to a variety of locations to interact with an assortment of colleagues. For others, the day may involve a series of appointments that take place in only one office where there is little contact with colleagues or friends. Regardless of the setting, the practice of psychotherapy is a satisfying endeavor accompanied by a number of rewards that are experienced by the majority of clinicians. A number of researchers have documented the most frequent benefits associated with clinical work, and below we summarize their findings.

Satisfaction of Helping

The most frequently endorsed occupational reward of psychotherapists is promoting growth in clients. Almost all (93%, to be exact) of us endorse it and experience it (Kramen-Kahn & Hansen, 1998).

The helper's high refers to the profound satisfaction of alleviating emotional distress and promoting personality growth in the lives of others. As a group, psychotherapists tend to be highly idealistic and altruistic, at least by their own report. They are motivated by a strong desire to help people, serve society, and improve the quality of life for those in distress (Guy, 1987; Guy, Poelstra, & Stark, 1989). In fact, this is the primary reason given by most psychotherapists for having chosen this career. Psychotherapists, with a few exceptions, are caring individuals willing to dedicate their lives to assisting others in emotional pain.

An old Chinese proverb reminds us:

If you want happiness for an hour—take a nap;
If you want happiness for a day—go fishing;
If you want happiness for a month—get married;
If you want happiness for a year—inherit a fortune; but
If you want happiness for a lifetime—help someone else.

There is no greater pleasure than knowing that you made a real, lasting difference in the life of another human being—a common experience for the effective psychotherapist, one that never loses its special meaning. To be present at the moment of significant insight or decision in the life of a client is a spiritual experience that connects the psychotherapist to the flow of life and creation, not unlike being present at the birth of a baby. This deep altruistic privilege, practically unknown in other professions, is derived from "being present at the ontic birth of a new being— assisting in its re-formation, definition, and extrusion" (Burton, 1972, p. 14). To participate in the restoration of another's soul, or the reestablishment of another's significant relationships, is what psychotherapists value above all other aims. As the Dakota say, "We will be known forever by the tracks we leave."

Such experiences serve as touchstones in our professional careers, as memories of transformative successes that are a source of comfort at times of self-doubt or discouragement. Every clinical trainee and graduate student knows that "this is what it's all about." Some veterans need to be reminded of this if they are to recapture the joy of clinical work.

We harbor a fantasy about helping colleagues vividly reexperience the collective privileges of being a mental health professional: each of us would create a videotape of some of our patients manifesting courageous behavioral changes and undergoing life transformations in which we were privileged to participate. Then we watch the montage of these former patients for 15 minutes every week: the loving child who on termination gives you a hug, a hand-crayoned picture, and the words "I love you"; the rebellious adolescent who began therapy by sitting mutely and staring defiantly at you but then completed treatment with gratitude and tears in his or her eyes; the lost young adult struggling to find an identity and relationship in the world and who did so with your assistance; the perennially battling couple who finally encountered each other and some marital happiness through the therapy work; the overwhelmed and working poor who found a resource in you and upon termination insisted that you accept a small token of their appreciation that you knew he or she could not really afford; the elderly client who resolved long-standing rifts in the family or made peace before death. The recovering alcoholic, the euthymic depressive, the sexual assault victim who completed treatment stronger than ever, the vulnerable who became more powerful. These strings of faces and voices would remind us that the vast majority of patients are assisted. The videotape montage would counterbalance the nagging images of those we have not helped, which tend to preoccupy our high-expectation brains.

Altruism gives back, its returns manifold in our careers and our lives. The Talmud teaches us, "A person possesses what he gives away." An Emily Dickinson (1890/2001) poem reminds us of its relationship to life satisfaction:

> If I can stop one heart from breaking,
> I shall not live in vain;
> If I can ease one life the aching,
> Or cool one pain,
> Or help one fainting robin
> Unto his nest again,
> I shall not live in vain.

Permanent Membership in the Client's World

Psychotherapy is often conducted intermittently throughout a patient's life. Those of us in practice for a number of years and remaining in one geographic location enjoy the experience of being "adopted" into the families of certain clients. Over time, we may see the same client for several distinctly separate courses of treatment. This lengthy relationship allows them to participate in more than just one moment of crisis. We psychotherapists get to join the client for her journey through life, witnessing and participating in the developmental milestones along the way (e.g., graduation, marriage, illness, child rearing, death of loved ones, aging).

When asked what we know now that we wished we learned in graduate school, one of our immediate answers is: Patients come back! And joyfully so.

Such long-term involvement and investment gives a deep sense of meaning to the caring psychotherapist who finds that her commitment to a particular individual is not easily surrendered at the time of the first termination. Periodic ongoing contact allows the clinician to have a lasting influence on the life and relationships. Although it can be difficult at times to wait to hear from a former client rather than initiating contact whenever she comes to mind, most psychotherapists are grateful for the occasional opportunity to hear from a favorite individual at a later point in her life journey.

Related to this is the opportunity to see other loved ones in treatment. It is not unusual for some psychotherapists to treat spouses, siblings, children, parents, or friends of current or former clients. This practice provides a meaningful participation in the world of clients, particularly when boundary concerns are ethically explicit and worked through with sensitivity and maturity.

Freedom and Independence

One of the most frequently mentioned benefits of the career is its freedom. Psychotherapists tend to be an independent, free-thinking cadre who value their intellectual independence. Independent of the work setting, we actually work for ourselves. Yes, we serve many people and may have a direct supervisor, but ultimately we answer to no one but ourselves. This independence is fiercely guarded, which may partially explain the deep resentment that exists toward managed care and peer review programs (Dumont, 1992).

As a rule, psychotherapists exercise considerable control over the total hours they work, number of days, and the hours of the day in the office. We can also control, or at least screen, the types of clients seen and the extent of professional involvements outside the practice of psychotherapy. This is particularly true of experienced practitioners, who by virtue of seniority are able to exercise choice in much of what they do. Private practitioners work for themselves; there is no other "boss."

The greater the degree of freedom experienced, the greater the amount of satisfaction reported, with those in independent practice expressing the greatest amount of satisfaction in virtually all studies (e.g., Boice & Myers, 1987; Norcross & Prochaska, 1983). Not surprisingly, therapists in mental health agencies report the least amount of freedom and corresponding job satisfaction.

Variety of Experiences

Related to the freedom and independence is the wide variety of experiences available to the therapist. As teenagers might say, psychotherapy is "an excellent adventure." One of our master therapists put it well:

> "I love the variety of people that I meet in this line of work. How else could I learn the personal stories of such interesting people? My therapy clients have included international spies, movie stars, scientists, politicians, and master thieves. I'd never meet these kinds of fascinating people in my life outside of the office."

Obviously, not every psychotherapist will treat stars and spies, but the reward persists. The opportunity to interact with a variety of individuals of different ages, educational levels, racial and ethnic backgrounds, and socioeconomic status affords the psychotherapist a ringside seat to the drama and intrigue of human existence. No two stories are alike, and no symptom complex is repeated the same way.

Psychotherapists who most value the emotional satisfactions derived from clinical practice expect to extend their careers well into their 70s (Guy, Stark, Poelstra, & Souder, 1987). Those who diversify their professional lives—and thus conduct fewer hours of therapy per week—are the most likely to plan for later retirement. It is so good that they want to prolong the rewards.

Doing therapy time and again with diverse clients opens us to a continual sense of wonder. The sheer variety allows us to renew our practice and ourselves. As with the diver who practices again and again but finds each dive is different, each patient and each session is a fresh opportunity with unique moments (Rosenbaum, 1999).

Intellectual Stimulation

In a unique way, the work of the psychotherapist is not unlike that of Sherlock Holmes. The search for the source of distress can take on the quality of careful detective work as the practitioner attempts to ascertain the etiology, development, and prognosis of a particular problem in the life of her patient. The search for the source of behavior change—what methods and relationships are likely to work for this patient in this context?—is equally challenging. Testing hypotheses, researching the literature for explanations, and experimenting with treatments are intellectually challenging. Simply put, we psychotherapists are immersed in the grandest and most complex of pursuits—the development and maintenance of the human mind (Yalom, 2002).

Psychotherapists tend to highly value the ongoing process of learning and increased understanding of human behavior that result from years of practice. We are interested in people, curious about human behavior, and committed to the process of discovery. As a result, the rich intellectual world associated with psychotherapy provides a virtual playground for the mind of the psychotherapist. Individuals of considerable intelligence are drawn to the career because of the degree of intellectual stimulation inherent in the work. Moreover, the screening process involved in the selection and training of psychotherapists typically limits entry to those of high intellectual ability.

Performing psychotherapy also facilitates acquisition of a related intellectual quality: wisdom, defined as expert knowledge in the fundamental pragmatics of life. One intriguing study (Smith, Staudinger, & Baltes, 1994) used think-aloud responses to wisdom-related dilemmas, such as a 28-year-old father facing unemployment within 3 months. Participants are asked to formulate a plan that covers what the father should do and consider in the next 3–5 years. Independent raters found psychotherapists' responses higher than those of other professionals on all five criteria of wisdom (factual knowledge, procedural knowledge, life span contextualism, value relativism, and management of uncertainty). Psychotherapists' elevated wisdom might be due to career selection, clinical training, or professional experiences, but, for whatever confluence of reasons, therapists have developed knowledge of life's pragmatics. We tend to think more deeply, complexly, and effectively about the human condition.

Emotional Growth

While stimulation of the intellect and acquisition of wisdom are considerable benefits of a career, psychotherapists accord more value to their own emotional growth. The vast majority of psychotherapists acknowledge experiencing emotional growth as a direct result of their professional work (Guy, Poelstra, & Stark, 1989). We prospect for ourselves; we find golden nuggets every day about ourselves, our feelings, and our histories.

The process of self-discovery begins in graduate school, where the future psychotherapist receives intensive supervision and training focused on both personality strengths and weaknesses. Trainees often enter their own psychotherapy at this point, to understand and master recurrent conflicts and interpersonal vulnerabilities. The commitment to ongoing emotional development becomes a lifelong passion, and periodic personal psychotherapy, supervision, and consultation continue across the career (Guy, Freudenberger, Farber, & Norcross, 1990).

Repeated encounters with diverse clients allow the therapist to confront and, we hope, master a variety of personal challenges. Over time, this process seems to increase the practitioner's own assertiveness, self-assurance, self-reliance, self-reflection, psychological mindedness, introspection, and sensitivity (Guy, 1987).

Experienced psychotherapists also find that there is much to be learned from and inspired by their clients, many of whom have insights or experiences that can be usefully applied to the psychotherapist's own life. The work changes us. In a study of patient-induced inspiration (Kahn & Harkavy-Friedman, 1997), practically all of the social workers surveyed had been inspired by their patients. Patients inspire us in their courage in overcoming obstacles and willingness to take chances, for two examples. And this inspiration leads, at least in some cases, to improvements in the therapist's thinking and behaviors outside of sessions (Kottler & Carlson, 2005). This is indeed a serendipitous benefit of our work, since the primary goal is the growth and development of the client.

Emotional growth assuredly encompasses the reward of self-knowledge. As every seasoned practitioner understands, self-knowledge is not a linear or uniformly pleasant experience. The more we strive for something bright, the more its dark counterpart is evident. As the psychotherapist tries to become more conscious and aware of him- or herself, the unconscious side is constellated more powerfully than that of the average person. The paradox is as follows: the more conscious a psychotherapist becomes, the more unconscious he or she becomes; the more light that is cast into a dark corner, the more the other corners appear dark (Guggenbuhl-Craig, 1971). The more one knows, the more one is aware of how little he/she knows. Self-knowledge *and* humility emerge as rewards of conducting psychotherapy.

Part of the self-knowledge and emotional growth of the psychotherapist resides in increased psychological mindedness (Guy & Brown, 1992). This core ability to reflect on the meaning and motivation of the self and others is enhanced by graduate training, professional socialization, and then years of clinical practice. Over the course of a career, ever increasing psychological mindedness depends on our appreciation of the intricacies of human feelings and behaviors. One typical result is a heightened sensitivity to the feelings of others, a greater comfort with the full spectrum of human emotions (Mahoney, 2003).

Reinforcement for Personality Qualities

The work of the psychotherapist provides a context within which to exercise and enjoy some of the very personality characteristics that are valued by the therapist (Guy, 1987). For example, most therapists enjoy conversation. They are comfortable talking about meaningful feelings and ideas. It is very reinforcing to discover that their ability to converse can bring relief and comfort. Psychotherapists as a rule are also good listeners. They enjoy encouraging others to talk and to relate meaningful experiences. The ability to comprehend the client's many nuances of meaning brings pleasure to the clinician, who habitually finds that being heard and prized contributes to the client's self-understanding and treatment success.

Psychotherapists are relational beings, probably more so than most other humans. The heart of enlightenment involves being together. The heart of suffering, by contrast, involves being apart, imprisoned in self-preoccupation and disconnectedness (Rosenbaum, 1999). Psychotherapy provides a relational opportunity to worship, to celebrate our fundamental and energizing interdependence (Orlinsky, 2005). There are moments in therapy when this energy and human beauty meet, and, when they meet, a healing influence resonates in all directions. We are all changed—and improved—by the work.

Psychotherapy also cultivates and reinforces the therapist's ability to tolerate intimacy, a common characteristic among most therapists. An abiding motivation for psychotherapists entering the profession is that it affords the opportunity to build meaningful connections. The ability to maintain intimacy enables the psychotherapist to journey into the private corners of clients' lives and uncover secrets often hidden from everyone else. We are cradlers of secrets (Yalom, 2002). We walk alongside clients, regardless of their radiating pain and trauma, in a journey toward health. The connection, the interdependence, is a powerful reward of clinical work.

There are many other personality qualities typical of mental health professionals that engender satisfaction and that are self-reinforcing in their own right. In other words, for many of us, the practice of psychotherapy permits us to be successful and effective while being ourselves. Many of us have found a comfortable fit that capitalizes on our interests and strengths.

As a final example, psychotherapists typically appreciate the ironies and paradoxes inherent in human existence. The tragicomic, absurd nature of the experiences of life are recognized by most therapists, who enjoy laughing and finding some element of humor in nearly everything. Such humor and irony in clinical practice are genuine sources of enjoyment. Several of our master therapists reported that humor was a constant companion in their self-care. As one master clinician suggests:

"This kind of work is very depressing, and one could easily become consumed by the upsetting and depressing events in the lives of our clients. So, even when I am working with a client, I might look for ways to lighten what is otherwise a very serious situation by adding a certain perspective to it that helps both the client and myself realize that there may be some parts of the situation that are not devastating. That way we both can get a chuckle out of it."

Another put it this way:

"It can be humorous that people are as difficult as they are. And then it's humorous that as therapists we think they shouldn't be so difficult. In fact, it's humorous to think that people should be any other way than what they are!"

REWARDS AWAY FROM THE OFFICE

The benefits of psychotherapeutic practice outlined above were largely limited to those experienced by the psychotherapist during a typical workday with patients. It is reassuring to know that there are plenty of good reasons for entering and remaining in this career. But it is not enough for us to know that we have found a suitable endeavor that helps others and fits us. We also hope that our vocational choice will benefit our relationships and our personal lives. Fortunately, research and experience confidently tell us that this is the case for psychotherapists.

Interpersonal Relationships

Because of the emotional growth that occurs as a result of practicing psychotherapy, it's not surprising that therapists regularly report that their ability to relate to a spouse or significant other is enhanced by their work (Guy, 1987; Weiss & Weiss, 1992). What might enhance therapists' relationships and marriages? Therapists say, in descending order, acceptance of their own part in marital/family problems (87% agreement), development of communication skills (85%), greater appreciation of their own marital/family strengths (85%), and greater acceptance of the spouse's/family's problems (84%) (Wetchler & Piercy, 1986). These qualities of acceptance, communication, and patience make therapists more flexible and accommodating to a spouse, increasing the degree of satisfaction attained from the relationship. Therapists commonly report that these benefits are the positive consequences of years of clinical practice.

Interestingly, the limited extant research has not confirmed that psychotherapists actually enjoy a higher level of marital satisfaction than the general population (e.g., Guy, Poelstra, & Stark, 1989; Wahl, Guy, & Brown, 1993). Couples with one or more therapists within the dyad have about the same quality or adjustment as couples without a therapist—with one big exception. If psychotherapists rated themselves as exhibiting high ability in conducting marital therapy, then their marriages were better. That is, self-rated ability as a marital therapist correlates significantly with marital quality (Murstein & Mink, 2004). It appears that simply being a psychotherapist does not improve a marriage, but being a (self-rated) expert does.

In a similar vein, psychotherapists routinely state that their relationships with other loved ones are aided by the growth and experiences associated with clinical practice. For example, nearly three-fourths of therapists surveyed in one of our studies noted that their work positively impacted their relationships with their children (Guy, Poelstra, & Stark, 1989). Children of psychotherapists, likewise, feel that certain skills of their parents—empathy, tolerance, expertise in handling problems, in particular—are of benefit to them (Golden & Farber, 1998). Despite jokes to the contrary, most psychotherapists believe they are better suited for parenting because of their professional knowledge and experience. Moreover, therapists' flexible schedules and high autonomy may allow them to be more available at times of illness or special need (Weiss & Weiss, 1992). Obviously, this is not always the case, but many clinicians are able to adjust their schedules to fit family needs.

Multitudes of psychotherapists credit their clinical training, personal psychotherapy, and professional experience with enabling them to intervene and disrupt established patterns within their family of origin in a helpful, even therapeutic, manner. Their personal growth and professional skills equipped them to confront family conflicts that were otherwise overwhelming.

An exemplar in this regard is Murray Bowen's (1972) pioneering work on changing his own family of origin. Bowen was part of a large extended kin group that had dominated a small southern town for many generations. Bowen intentionally intruded into most of the dominant triangles of his immediate family by means of a surprising strategy. He sent off letters that told various relatives about the unpleasant gossip that others were circulating about them. He signed these letters with such endearing salutations as "Your Meddlesome Brother" or "Your Strategic Son." He also preannounced an impending visit. Bowen then arrived, as heralded, to deal with the predictably indignant reactions of his relatives. The effect on the family was dramatic. Many previously closed-off relationships were reopened. Once the initial fury against Bowen had subsided, his intervention created a warm climate of better feelings all around.

In a similar vein, psychotherapists relate that their experience as practitioners improves the climate and quality of their friendships (e.g., Cogan, 1977; Guy, Poelstra, & Stark, 1989). Why? As before, the therapists' emotional growth, comfort with intimacy, and communication skills enhance their ability to maintain meaningful friendships. The increased understanding and acceptance resulting from clinical practice probably also make us more accepting and supportive.

We speculate—but are unaware of any research on the matter—that conducting psychotherapy modifies a therapist's interpersonal priorities. After working daily with people suffering horrid abuses, staggering losses, and unremitting conflicts, our own relational squabbles are often transformed into relatively mundane annoyances. After sessions with parents who have just lost their young children, it would seem petty to go home and complain that we would have preferred a different color in the new toaster! We become more appreciative of what we have and more supportive of those around us. The work *does* change us!

Personal Effectiveness

These encouraging reports of enhanced relationships converge with psychotherapists' convictions that their work has improved their life effectiveness. Practicing psychotherapy summons forth a wide array of cognitive, emotional, and behavioral skills useful for confronting the dilemmas and transitions of life. For example, insights about compatibility and communication gained by assisting clients certainly are useful to the psychotherapist when selecting a partner, deciding to have children, adjusting to relocation, or struggling to raise a family. Assisting a client with the grief and pain resulting from the loss of a loved one provides valuable experience in facing similar personal losses due to divorce, the departure of children, or the death of a friend. The ability to confront one's own mortality, aging, and eventual death is influenced by the opportunity to experience these events vicariously in the lives of clients.

One of our master therapists describes his gratitude in this way:

> "I have learned so much about life through the experiences of my clients. They have changed me, and I'm a better person for having been a part of their struggles and pain. I've lived several lifetimes and viewed life through the eyes of literally hundreds of people. This can't help but improve my own chances for a happy life."

The empirical research comparing the personal lives of practicing psychologists and research psychologists is supportive of this message as well. Consistent with the literature to be reviewed in the next chapter, the clinicians suffer more anxiety, depression, and emotional exhaustion than the researchers. However, the clinicians are more satisfied with their lives and more likely to feel that their work has influenced them in positive ways (Radeke & Mahoney, 2000). Specifically, clinicians experience a surfeit of personal benefits: their work has made them wiser and more aware, increased their capacity to enjoy life, improved their value system, and accelerated their psychological development (Radeke & Mahoney, 2000). The ability to take what has been learned by assisting others in negotiating life challenges and applying it to one's own life may well be one of the most unheralded rewards of psychotherapeutic practice.

Life Meaning

We rarely hear our therapist colleagues complain that their lives lack meaning. On the contrary, life as a therapist is filled with purpose and meaning, a life of service in which we daily transcend our personal wishes and turn our gaze toward the needs and growth of the other (Yalom, 2002). The threads merge into a deeper meaning or life mission.

We will have (much) more to say about mission as a means of alleviating distress and renewing passion in Chapter 11. For now, we would highlight the point by noting that psychotherapy offers rewards in terms of mission and meaning that few professions offer. Our professional concerns are never irrelevant to the most important things in life. Psychotherapists have a transcendent purpose or mission beyond ourselves. It almost seems greedy to request or expect more from a profession.

Public Recognition

It is a standing joke in southern California that a psychotherapist "lives on every block." This perception may also be expressed in other parts of the country, such as New York City, Chicago, and Boston. However, in most localities there is sufficient novelty associated with the role of psychotherapist to afford the profession a modicum of prestige and respect.

People usually acknowledge the considerable education, training, and emotional strength needed to conduct psychotherapy. Every therapist has heard patients sympathize with and praise them with such statements as "I could never do your job everyday!" The psychotherapist's role and the spiritually laden meaning of the role of "helper" combine in the mind of the observer to create the impression that the clinician is a special person of notable ability and personal worth. There is a mystique to the role that wins both the admiration of those who tend to idealize healers and the begrudging respect of those who may be suspicious of the "mind games" of therapists.

It is not unusual for psychotherapists to be consulted by family and friends as though we are psychic wizards privy to the secrets of human existence. How often have you been approached outside the office for advice on child-rearing, marital adjustment, or dream interpretation? As experts on human behavior, our opinions are typically given more influence and power than is warranted or even desired. Yes, it can lead to some embarrassing moments. But, let's be honest: on the whole, while a bit disconcerting at times, the prestige associated with being a "mind healer" is enjoyable and appreciated when kept within reasonable bounds.

Employment Opportunities

Competent psychotherapists are in demand in most parts of the country for their services. In addition to conducting psychotherapy, clinicians are often welcomed to teach at local churches, synagogues, PTAs, colleges, and high schools. Hospitals, nursing homes, residential treatment facilities, and community programs are eager to have mental health professionals involved or consulting. Publishers are always interested in a clinician's manuscript or article. The media seek the opinion or advice of the prominent practitioner. It does not take long to discover that this is a highly marketable career. Even in areas smothered by managed care and governmental cutbacks, the career opportunities available to talented psychotherapists are limited only by a lack of imagination.

The diversity of professional activities and variety of employment settings are definite assets. Psychotherapists appreciate the high degree of flexibility regarding work setting, schedule, professional labor, and income (Gottfredson, 1987). As mentioned previously, the psychotherapist ultimately works for herself. The neophyte clinician entering a highly competitive marketplace should take heart: over time, an increasing number of career opportunities will become available.

And, despite evolving economic conditions, a career in psychotherapy provides a comfortable income. In most cases, psychotherapists earn an annual income well above the average of the general population. We can also supplement primary means of income through a variety of part-time options, as noted above. The profession is not as financially lucrative as it once was, but most agree that the compensation continues to be adequate to support those already in practice and to attract those considering careers in psychotherapy.

INTERNALIZING REWARDS
AND REORIENTING ACCORDINGLY

It is easy to recognize and celebrate the rewards of practicing psychotherapy. We can recapture that precious sense of wonder, awe, and reverence for evolving lives and unfolding mysteries. Even as we shovel the snow, we can appreciate the wonder of each snowflake.

Perhaps this chapter has simply confirmed your own sense of why you chose to become a psychotherapist. You may have identified many occupational privileges among the list that you are already enjoying. On the other hand, perhaps you were surprised to note some benefits that you have yet to encounter. A review of this list can serve as a focal point, as you consider ways to maximize the rewards.

However, we must do more then simply recognize the occupational privileges. We must internalize them as means of self-care and replenishment. We must build in a way to count our blessings. We recommend the weekly imagery exercise on therapeutic successes previously mentioned. Or a few moments every week sitting quietly and being infused with a career of healing and a life of meaning. Or a gratitude journal, a fashionable method of positive psychology, in which you record daily or weekly several things for which you are thankful.

One of our master clinicians simply said: "I have a great love for what I do. When the job gets stressful, I focus on how much I love the work." And one of our workshop participants writes:

"After each session, I write down the things that went well. This allows me to focus on the positive and to learn what is most helpful for my clients. In the past I tried to ruminate over what went wrong and blame myself for it. This new approach has proved very beneficial for both the client and myself."

The specific method should be tailored to your preferences, of course, but we implore you to internalize the rewards on a regular basis as one antidote to the inevitable hazards of conducting psychotherapy (reviewed in the next chapter). The lack of therapeutic success is typically cited as the single most stressful feature of conducting therapy; almost 75% of practitioners complain of it (Farber & Heifetz, 1982). Like most achievement-oriented graduate school victims, we selectively obsess on failures and thereby neglect the process and success of so much of psychotherapy. We need to counterbalance our preoccupation with the failures by recognizing our successes, internalizing the rewards, and relishing them.

The accumulating research on psychotherapists' professional experiences boils down to "feeling blessed" (in an emotional rather than theological sense) and "feeling burdened" dimensions (Orlinsky & Rønnestad, 2005). The two are only slightly correlated ($r = -.13$) and thus independent dimensions. About 20% of therapists feel highly blessed but also heavily burdened, a mixed quality of life. But the largest group of therapists—about 40%—score high on blessed and low on burdened. They experience a fulfilled life.

The chapters that follow in this volume will identify an assortment of skillful attitudes and methods to master the hazards of clinical practice and, more importantly, to thrive in your self-care. Many of these methods will involve enhancements of the rewards described in this chapter. Psychotherapists have compelling evidence to be optimistic about enjoying the benefits ascribed to our healing profession. The work *does* change us, frequently for the better.

SELF-CARE CHECKLIST

✓ Recall that career satisfaction among psychotherapists is consistently high and rivals (or exceeds) that of other professionals.

✓ Remember your reasons for entering the profession in the first place as a means of refreshing your sense of calling and professional fulfillment.

✓ Build into your weekly schedule a concrete method to count your blessings, such as an imagery exercise or a gratitude journal.

✓ Attend to the profound satisfaction of helping others; vividly recall the life-transforming psychotherapies in which you were privileged to participate.

✓ Look for ways to create a greater sense of freedom and independence in your work.

✓ Variety and intellectual stimulation are indispensable. What can you do to increase their impact on your schedule and professional duties?

✓ Satisfaction from helping others is crucial, so be sure to include at least some clinical activities that demonstrate you are helping someone!

✓ Enjoy maintaining relationships with clients that span years, even decades, involving intermittent courses of treatment.

✓ Your work will ideally capitalize on both your natural and acquired abilities. Do what you do well.

✓ A sense of humor and the absurd is one of your most potent stress relievers. Practice!

✓ Be careful when applying your expertise to your family of origin . . . fools rush in where angels fear to tread.

✓ Self-monitor the quality of your friendships. Do they sustain you?

✓ Remember: you are actually self-employed, regardless of who you work for. Maintaining this perspective brings great freedom of choice.

✓ Clinical practice may not make you rich, but if it is your calling, it is a wonderful way to make a living.

✓ Bear in mind, particularly during your beleaguered moments, that there are typically many more benefits than hazards associated with the practice of psychotherapy.

RECOMMENDED READING

Coster, J. S., & Schwebel, M. (1997). Well-functioning in professional psychologists. *Professional Psychology: Research and Practice, 28*, 5–13.

Goldberg, C. (1992). *The seasoned psychotherapist—triumph over adversity.* New York: Norton.

Kottler, J. A., & Carlson, J. (Eds.). (2005). *The client who changed me: Stories of therapist personal transformation.* New York: Routledge.

CHAPTER 3

Recognizing the Hazards

with Joan Laidig

> It almost looks as if analysis were the third of those "impossible" professions in which one can be sure beforehand of achieving unsatisfying results. The other two, which have been known much longer, are education and government.

Thus wrote Freud (1937/1964) in *Analysis Terminable and Interminable*. The lack and uncertainty of therapeutic success is typically cited as the single most stressful feature of conducting therapy. Almost 75% of practitioners highlight it as a significant hazard (Farber & Heifetz, 1982).

So, let us begin by saying it aloud: practicing psychotherapy is often a demanding and grueling enterprise. Freud correctly characterized it as an "impossible" profession. Mental health professionals are regularly engulfed by their clients' pain and disability, are routinely confronted by conscious and unconscious hostility, and are ethically bound to secrecy about the most troubling confessions and occasionally the most heinous of crimes. All of this is accomplished under unremitting pressure in frequently less than humane working conditions with interpersonally disturbed patients. Emotional depletion, physical isolation, and psychic withdrawal seem natural responses. Throw in the inescapable disruptions to our personal lives and one is tempted to accept the dramatic assertion that "If we ever really considered the possible risks in getting involved with a client, we would not do so for any price. Never mind that we will catch their colds and flus, what about their pessimism, negativity, and psychopathology" (Kottler, 1986, p. 8).

Psychotherapist self-care begins with recognizing and preparing for the inevitable hazards of the undertaking. Understanding its various liabilities demystifies the process and enables us to effectively cope with its downside. Those who understand the etiology and impact of these liabilities are most effective in minimizing their negative consequences, and thus more successfully "leave it at the office" at the end of a long workday.

Table 3.1 offers a summary of the most prominent hazards associated with clinical work. This nonexhaustive list of stressors is culled from the vast literature on the topic, which interestingly enough is at least twice the size of the literature on the benefits of clinical work. Please minimize your exposure to this frightening list, lest you stare at it for hours and put in for early retirement! In actuality, we believe a little stress inoculation is effective, and, in any case, we will not get to all of the items in the listing.

In this chapter we have set for ourselves the ambitious task of summarizing the vast literature on psychotherapist stress and extracting its recurrent themes. Our integration begins by reviewing six overlapping burdens rooted in practice itself—physical isolation, emotional isolation, patient behaviors, working conditions, therapeutic relationships, and the industrialization of mental health—and then a series of interactive hazards centered on the person of the psychotherapist—motivations for becoming a therapist, the fusion of work stress and therapist personality, and intercurrent life events. We conclude with multiple methods to anticipate, master, and, when necessary, accept these hazards.

PHYSICAL ISOLATION

Few rookies are prepared for the gnawing effects of physical isolation on their inner world. The need for complete privacy with no interruptions is simply accepted as a requirement for conducting psychotherapy's private journey. Isolation is regarded as essential in order to provide the context needed for in-depth exploration. But, however necessary it may be, isolation comes at a price. The paradox of being so alone in the midst of this most intimate of interpersonal encounters is perhaps one of the least understood hazards of psychotherapy (Guy & Liaboe, 1986; Hellman, Morrison, & Abramowitz, 1986).

In contrast to the camaraderie and teamwork characteristic of clinical training, the practice of psychotherapy over the course of a career is basically a solitary task. While some therapists participate in treatment teams and cotherapy, most clinicians are forced by economics of time and

TABLE 3.1. Prominent Hazards Encountered in Conducting Psychotherapy

Patient behaviors

Hostile transference
Suicidal statements and attempts
Anger toward therapist
Severe depression
Apathy, lack of motivation
Premature termination
Passive–aggressive behavior
(withdrawing, withholding)
Being sued for malpractice
Patient violence (assault, threat, attacks)
Terminally ill patients
Severe resistance
Dependent personality

Working conditions

Organizational politics
Managed care
Onerous paperwork
Excessive workload
Scheduling constraints
Work overinvolvement
High expectations
Compliance with excessive rules and
regulations
Exclusion from administrative decisions
Low salary
Paucity of secretarial help
Time pressures and deadlines
Colleague misbehavior
Resistance to new ideas in agencies

Emotional depletion

Boredom
Physical exhaustion/fatigue
Difficulty in leaving "psychodynamics"
at the office
Inevitable need to relinquish patients
Constraints of the "50-minute hour"
Identifying with the patient's
psychopathology
Compassion fatigue/secondary
traumatization
Repeated emotional strain
Lack of therapeutic success
Doubts about career choice
Activation of preexisting
psychopathology

Psychic isolation

Professional competition
Maintaining confidentiality
Withholding personal information
Setting aside personal concerns
One-way intimacy
Controlling emotions
Idealization and omnipotence
Devaluation and attack
Public perceptions
Physical isolation from the world and
from colleagues
Physical inactivity and fatigue

Therapeutic relationships

Responsibility for patients
Difficulty in working with disturbed
patients
Lack of gratitude from patients
Countertransferential feelings
Developing a pathological orientation
Loss of authenticity in dealing with
clients

Personal disruptions

Financial concerns
Illness and disability
Aging and retirement
Loss/death of loved one or family
member
Divorce
Marriage
Pregnancy
Parenthood
Relocation
Departure of children
Terminal illness

Miscellaneous stressors

Idealistic criteria for client treatment
outcome
Monotony of work
Difficulty in evaluating progress
Doubts about the efficacy of
psychotherapy

money to go it alone. Treatment is typically provided by a single therapist who works throughout the day in consecutive sessions interspersed with occasional breaks. Short of considerable effort, the practitioner moves throughout her day alone, with minimal contact with associates. For those in hospital or clinic environments, group meetings and in-service workshops provide interruptions in the physical isolation. For those in private practice, even when associated with a larger group, there are few breaks in the physical isolation of the typical workday. It comes as no surprise that isolation is a leading complaint of experienced independent practitioners (Tryon, 1983).

It logically follows that physical isolation from friends and family also characterizes the practice of psychotherapy. We all know that most psychotherapists cannot be reached during a therapy session. Some have joked that even God cannot reach the dedicated clinician without an appointment! Although access can be gained in an emergency, the more serendipitous, casual contacts by friends and family during a workday are quite limited. Visitors cannot stop by for an unscheduled greeting or lunch. Friends cannot call during sessions to share a few moments of contact.

Even more unusual is the deficient access to news of daily local, national, and international events. Since our primary or even exclusive interpersonal contact is limited to therapy clients, it is possible to remain uninformed of recent events. Unless a client announces an assassination, military initiative, or natural catastrophe, it may be hours before we learn of a major event. One of our master therapists related the following illustrative story:

> "I had a full schedule of consecutive clients on the day that the United Nations forces attacked Iraq. I had no idea what had happened until several hours later, when a client mentioned it as she walked in for her session with a television in hand for us both to watch. Needless to say, I was surprised at her news, and I had to smile at the irony that my three previous clients had not thought it was appropriate, or a good use of their time, to inform me that U.S. military forces had attacked another country!"

Such occurrences are the rule: what happens in the world outside of the office is oddly separate from the world inside the therapy session.

The isolation of the consulting room and the paucity of physical movement can lead to an unusual kind of environmental deprivation. Therapists report struggling with sleepiness or recurrent daydreams while trying to concentrate on clinical material. Even the content of the sessions themselves can develop a numbing similarity, causing a mental dullness to creep over us during the course of a long day. Therapists may begin to treat all clients in parallel ways using similar techniques and similar words. Eventually, the authenticity and creativity of the therapist become circumscribed (Freudenberger & Robbins, 1979). The result is a clinician who fulfills her role mechanically, producing a sense of boredom and isolation.

Conducting a therapy session involves relatively little physical activity. Many therapists sit for 8 or more hours a day in the same chair and room, rendering them physically exhausted from immobilization (Will, 1979). We rarely walk, stretch, or exercise. Such sedentary days suppress physical releases of stress after continued exposure to emotional pain. The research indicates that those who do not take time out from their busy schedules to exercise and participate in outside activities are more likely to suffer from fatigue and emotional exhaustion (e.g., Hoeksema, Guy, Brown, & Brady, 1993).

EMOTIONAL ISOLATION

Unfortunately, therapist isolation is not limited to the physical realm. The isolation pervades our psyches. Despite the intense relational contact of psychotherapy, many practitioners feel alone emotionally. One study (Thoreson, Miller, & Krauskopf, 1989) revealed that 8% of the psychologists reported significant distress during the preceding year due to recurrent feelings of loneliness.

The exclusive focus on our patients' psychological world leaves little room for the expression of the clinician's feelings and needs, particularly as they relate to her life. The role of the psychotherapist requires a self-imposed limitation on self-disclosure. The criterion becomes "what is in the best interests of the client." Even in the most active treatments, clinicians exercise considerable restraint in keeping feelings hidden. We, as clinicians, set aside the personal concerns of the day, such as disputes with loved ones, financial problems, or even an upset stomach, in order to focus on the client—even when our own worries seem more serious than the patient's.

The therapeutic process further requires a great deal of emotional discipline on the part of the practitioner. We need to mute or restrain feelings in the name of competent treatment. And psychotherapists do experience strong emotions in their work: in one study, approximately 80% of therapists experienced fear, anger, and sexual feelings in the context of their work (Pope & Tabachnick, 1993). The constant emotional regulation isolates the therapist from others and possibly from her own feelings.

Patients' reactions to the clinician compound the psychic isolation (Freudenberger, 1990a). For example, overly idealizing the therapist hinders attempts at a genuine encounter. Therapists can become burdened with unrealistic expectations that leave them little room to be themselves (Goldberg, 1986). Even worse, some therapists actually accept client idealization as warranted, leading to a sense of omnipotence that isolates them from their true feelings. In other cases, devaluing and attacking the therapist can result in their feeling discouraged, humiliated, or rejected. In fact, competent treatment may require that therapists absorb these projections rather than defend against them.

The ethical and legal requirements of confidentiality result in a tendency for psychotherapists to split off the emotional impact of their work from the rest of life (Spiegel, 1990). While many practitioners seek emotional support from family and friends to alleviate feelings of alienation, the confidentiality requirement impedes using such support except in certain instances (Tamura, Guy, Brady, & Grace, 1994). Therapists must monitor closely any self-disclosure of their workday to avoid inadvertent domestic violations of confidentiality, making the venting of frustration or the sharing of a therapeutic success a complicated matter (Spiegel, 1990).

Such secrecy conflicts with the need for open communication among family members (Kaslow & Schulman, 1987). The family may perceive confidentiality as a rule that shuts them out from the therapist's world, engendering jealousy and resentment from those who might otherwise help ease the isolation. Is there a psychotherapist alive who has not experienced the disheartening duplicity of one moment being the attentive, empathic psychotherapist and the next moment the tired, preoccupied family member (Brady, Healy, Norcross, & Guy, 1995)?

All these factors converge and contribute to the "one-way" intimacy of conducting psychotherapy (Guy, 1987). The client is asked to share herself in great detail, while the clinician responds with little disclosure. Thus, the therapist experiences a sense of intimacy with many people, but with little personal risk or expressed vulnerability; true mutuality is lacking. Often the seasoned veteran has no one with whom to share deeply meaningful moments in the private journey of a psychotherapy client. The more intense the psychotherapy-related experience, the more difficult and unnatural it becomes to withhold it from a loved one. Therapists wind up habitually suppressing intense feelings, leaving them unprocessed and unresolved.

Since the treatment contract requires that the relationship eventually end, psychotherapists find that they are in the business of saying repeated good-byes to individuals they have come to value. The cumulative effects of these terminations on the emotional life of psychotherapists are just beginning to be understood (e.g., Guy & Brown, 1993; Guy, French, Poelstra, & Brown, 1993). Some find it difficult to let go of these meaningful relationships, particularly when they have been the source of considerable satisfaction and meaning (Brady, Guy, Poelstra, & Brown, 1996). The hurt is often a private loss unvoiced and unshared with friends. Over time, these repeated losses can beget reluctance to attach, to a disinclination to care deeply. We hate to lose contact with some patients; we miss them, we think about them periodically, and we wonder whether they will initiate contact with us again. Planned terminations are necessary losses and a legitimate source of mourning endemic to the profession.

Even relationships with colleagues can have an isolating component in them. Therapists have a strong desire to appear emotionally stable and clinically expert to peers (Guy, Poelstra, & Stark, 1989). The increased competition for patients and referrals associated with managed care adds fuel to the perceived need to always be at the top of your game. "Top Gun" rivalries—therapists competing with one another in a hostile manner—can become common (Persi, 1992). It is difficult for clinicians to share concerns openly if they perceive that doing so might put their livelihood and professional standing at risk.

Rivalry and resultant isolation often follow from ideological schisms. Raised and socialized in a "dogma eat dogma" environment that pits one theoretical orientation against another (Norcross & Goldfried, 2005), therapists tend to avoid colleagues of differing persuasions and professions. Divisions between, say, psychoanalysts and behaviorists, or psychopharmacologists and psychotherapists, generate the ironic feeling of being alone among colleagues.

Male psychotherapists typically experience even more difficulty cultivating relationships with peers, since most men are socialized to inhibit expression of most emotions and to interact competitively with other men, thereby avoiding emotional closeness with male colleagues (Brooks, 1990). Their disinclination toward emotional support and honest communication may perpetuate relationships among men characterized by competition and homophobia. All told, secrecy inhibits sharing among colleagues and breeds loneliness.

Finally, some psychotherapists find it difficult to set aside the interpretive observer role when leaving the office (Zur, 1993). While at home they may find that the practiced restraint and reflective treatment posture make it difficult for them to be themselves. Such detached expertise hinders the therapist from responding in a genuine, spontaneous way, leading to artificial interactions (Freudenberger & Robbins, 1979; Guy, 1987). In short, it is difficult to leave the psychodynamics at the office and "turn off" the therapeutic role while at home.

This loss of spontaneity and genuineness may make the therapist seem aloof outside of the office. Family and friends may find it difficult to get us to self-disclose. Worse still, the emotional depletion after a long, exhausting day may kill any motivation for the therapist to reach out and make emotional contact with loved ones. Instead, she may withdraw and remain isolated, even when physically surrounded by those who wish to interact. Emotional isolation is more frequently reported by inexperienced clinicians who have not yet mastered the skill of removing the "therapeutic mask."

PATIENT BEHAVIORS

Our colleague Gerry Koocher (1999), who works with children and families confronting life-threatening illnesses, has written movingly of his work-related nightmares. One recurrent dream is that Gerry is in line for a roller-coaster theme park.

> As the line winds down slowly toward the start of the ride, I notice that I'm standing among friends, relatives, and dozens of bald-headed or bewigged children, several of whom I recognize as patients I treated before they died from cancer. Suddenly we are on the leading platform, and I notice a sign with large red letters: "WARNING! Up to 40 percent of riders fall to their deaths. Check your safety bar." I find myself seated in the last seat of the back car. I pull the safety bar toward me and hear a reassuring "click," as it snaps into place. As I look up the car begins to roll down the chute, and I notice that many of the riders in front of me have not secured their belts. I feel a desperate urge to reach out and help, but am locked in my seat and cannot help. We plunge into darkness that is broken by the flash of a strobe light. With each flash I see more empty seats in front of me. There is nothing I can do. (Koocher, 1999, p. 25)

This disturbing dream encapsulates what many psychotherapists feel when they are unable to reach a patient or when a patient disappears, dies, or suicides. One need not be an expert on dream interpretation to see that our rational desires to help and comfort are trumped in sleep by the magical wish to cure everyone and to stave off death. The dream powerfully reminds us of the stressful contacts and despairing lives that some patients share with us. We try to insulate ourselves from such disappointments, but some losses are like sandpaper on the soul.

Psychotherapists work with emotionally distressed and conflict-ridden patients. The natural consequence is that we rarely see people "at their best" (Guy, 1987). Dealing exclusively with pathological populations begins to color our perceptions of society and humanity. For instance, a clinician who works with sexual abuse victims day after day can easily form a skewed perspective of the world (Pearlman & Saakvitne, 1995). Continual immersion in a world suffused with psychopathology and dysfunction isolates the clinician and constitutes an occupational hazard (Freudenberger & Robbins, 1979).

Not only are we as susceptible to clients' contagious emotions as anybody else, but we also possess certain vulnerabilities unique to the profession (Schwartz, 2004)—a double whammy of sorts. We are supposed to be perfect—empathic, mature, selfless, kind, hopeful, and wise—no matter how the client is. Despite intense provocations on the client's part, we are supposed to avoid pejorative remarks, wisecracks, or bitter complaints to the person/patient precipitating our distress. An impossible profession, indeed!

Most empirical research on the stressors of psychotherapy practice has been conducted on specific client behaviors. In general (e.g., Deutsch, 1984; Farber, 1983a; Kramen-Kahn & Hansen, 1998), specific patient presentations found to be the most distressing are suicidal statements and acts, aggression toward the therapist, severely depressed patients, premature termination, profound apathy, and the loss of a patient. Let us consider these and other patient behaviors in turn.

Of all the patients who test our patience, the suicidal top the list (e.g., Chemtob, Bauer, Hamada, Pelowski, & Muraoka, 1989). Jeffrey Kottler (1986) describes the challenge of treating suicidal patients on four levels. First, therapists may feel terrified at the knowledge of being so close to someone so desperate that nothingness seems like a viable option. Second, therapists feel immense responsibility to help a suicidal patient. The moral and professional obligations are extraordinary, and any mistake may prove to be lethal. Third, once a patient is assessed as suicidal, the entire therapeutic process is altered. Extra precautions on the part of the staff must be made, and everything must be done "by the book." The margin for error is small, and the pressure on the therapist profound (Kottler, 1986, p. 74). Fourth, it is particularly difficult to leave the problems of dealing with a suicidal patient "at the office."

The probabilities of mental health trainees and professionals having a patient commit suicide are fairly high, sad to say. More than one-quarter of psychologists and one-half of psychiatrists will experience a patient's suicide (Chemtob et al., 1989). More than one in four interns/trainees will encounter a patient suicide attempt, and at least one in nine will experience a completed patient suicide (Brown, 1987; Kleespies, Penk, & Forsyth, 1993).

In the event of a patient suicide, the psychotherapists involved will probably experience substantial disruptions in their personal and professional lives. One-third of psychotherapists who experienced a patient's suicide subsequently suffer from severe mental distress (Hendin et al., 2004). Several factors contribute to the severe distress: failure to hospitalize an imminently suicidal patient who then died; a treatment decision the therapist felt contributed to the suicide; negative reactions from the therapist's institution; and/or fear of a lawsuit by the patient's relatives (Hendin et al., 2004). Trainees who experienced a patient suicide, as compared to trainees who had patients only express suicidal ideation, felt greater shock, disbelief, failure, sadness, self-blame, guilt, shame, and depression (Kleespies et al., 1993). Patient suicide may represent the ultimate failure for a psychotherapist, who is left to deal with sadness, anger, self-doubt, confusion, and the fear of its happening again. (The American Association of Suicidology has a Clinician Survivor Task Force to help practitioners who lose a patient to suicide; go to *mypage.iusb.edu/ ~jmcintos/basicinfo.htm.*)

Also high atop the lists of stressful patient behaviors is aggression. An early psychiatrist (Freeman, 1968, p. 286) declared dramatically that "the major occupational hazard of psychiatrists is being shot by former patients." No one agreed with him literally then or now, but his forceful statement underscored the wide prevalence of physical attacks, threats, and stalking directed at therapists.

Reviews of the literature reveal that nearly half of all psychotherapists are threatened, harassed, or physically attacked by a patient at some point in their careers (Guy, Brown, & Poelstra, 1992; Haller & Deluty, 1988; Pope & Tabachnick, 1993). Therapists are more likely to be attacked in hospitals and clinics than in private practices (Tyron, 1983). The most frequent negative effects of actual physical attacks are an increase in personal vulnerability, escalation of fearfulness, decrease in emotional well-being, increase in a loved one's concern for the clinician's personal safety, and diminution of perceived competence (Guy, Brown, & Poelstra, 1990a, 1990b, 1991). Intense anxiety, fatigue, headaches, hyperactivity, nightmares, flashbacks, and intermittent anger are also common consequences of patient violence (Guy et al., 1990a, 1990b; Wykes & Whittington, 1991). Those clinicians expressing the most worry were those who had been previously attacked, those working in hospitals, and those physically injured in prior patient assaults.

Patient aggression manifests itself even beyond overt physical attacks, of course. Unwanted phone calls to the home or office, verbal threats against one's personal safety and that of one's family, and threats of destruction to the office contents or home all represent violence (Guy et al., 1992). Approximately 5–15% of psychotherapists have been stalked by current or former clients (e.g., Gentile, Asamne, Harmell, & Weathers, 2002; Purcell, Powell, & Mullen, 2005; Romans, Hays, & White, 1996), largely motivated by anger or infatuation. An illustrative example: A female psychologist in private practice was forced to obtain two restraining orders against a former patient. The woman followed the therapist's car on numerous occasions, tried to stop her in the middle of the street, kept her home under surveillance, made telephone calls to other professionals defaming the psychologist, and made verbal and written threats.

Severely apathetic and depressed clients are bound to evoke anxiety in a psychotherapist. A continuous string of "uh," "um," "yes," or "no" can generate frustration in the best of us. A patient who is totally withdrawn and nearly silent can make a single hour seem endless; time seems to stand still. Eventually, therapists may begin to suspect that they must be doing something wrong. Sometimes, they even begin talking and answering for the client, in which case the whole process breaks down. Whenever this happens, the therapist feels under tremendous pressure to "get" the client to speak and make the treatment "work" (Corey & Corey, 1989).

Extensive work with trauma survivors, which involves listening to a litany of detailed descriptions of atrocities and constantly empathizing with clients, can also take a high toll on clinicians. Many experts believe that the most effective therapists ironically are also the most vulnerable to this hazard, as those who have the greatest capacity for empathy are at greatest risk for compassion fatigue (Miller, 1998). In this condition, described variously as vicarious traumatization (Pearlman & Saakvitne, 1995), compassion fatigue, or secondary traumatic stress (Figley, 1995), therapists repeatedly exposed to graphic trauma material via their clients' personal accounts can develop mild PTSD-like symptoms and experience changes in their frame of reference. Such distressing responses tend to be even more stressful to practitioners who (1) conduct a lot of treatment with survivors, (2) have a personal trauma history, and (3) endure higher levels of exposure to graphic details regarding sexual abuse (Brady, Guy, Poelstra, & Brokaw, 1999; Little & Hamby, 1996). Further, clients with histories of abuse or interpersonal violence are more likely to engage in self-destructive behaviors, dissociation, and acting out (Gamble, Pearlman, Lucca, & Allen, 1994). Trauma work produces a soul weariness that comes with caring.

Virtually all patients experiencing interpersonal difficulties will bring those problematic relationship patterns into the consulting room with them. Perhaps the patients who are most difficult to manage are those suffering from personality disorders. Passive–aggressive and covertly resistant behaviors, for example, are special challenges. The most notorious signs of passive–aggressiveness include late arrival, minimal disclosure, and a hollow assurance that all is well. Accentuating the distress is that these behaviors are so hard to deal with directly—they evince an "elusive" quality, not always amenable to firm evidence or confident interpretation.

A common passive–aggressive manifestation in psychotherapy is premature termination, which frequently results in relatively high levels of psychotherapist stress (Farber, 1983b). A meta-analysis of 125 studies (Wierzbicik & Pekarki, 1993) found that the average dropout rate for patients in mental health agencies is a whopping 47%! Many of our clients terminate before meeting their therapeutic goals, leaving us all feeling confused, uncertain, and disappointed with treatment outcome.

The ultimate test of stress management may well involve patients suffering from borderline personality disorder. In one person, the therapist may encounter scores of distressing patient behaviors: recurrent suicidal threats, self-mutilating acts, intense anger alternating with chronic dysphoria, identity disturbance, vicarious exposure to trauma material, and the worst elements of histrionic and passive–aggressive disorders. The therapist may be so busy extinguishing weekly brushfires attributable to "acting-out" behavior that attending to the underlying forest fire in the patient's identity may go undone. Patients suffering from borderline traits and other characterological disorders are also prone to litigation.

The threat of malpractice or ethical complaint is omnipresent in health care professions, and psychotherapy is no exception. Approximately 10–12% of mental health practitioners will need to respond to a licensing complaint during their careers, all the more so if you are male and a psychiatrist. But only about 2% of practitioners end up being a defendant in a malpractice suit during their careers (e.g., Dorken, 1990; Pope & Vasquez, 2005; Schoenfeld, Hatch, & Gonzalez, 2001). The prevalence is rising but it is important to remember that it is still relatively low.

We suffer from not only an actual lawsuit but also the potential risk of such a suit. The threat of malpractice can paralyze us and cause us to practice too defensively. Lawyers and risk managers repeatedly warn us to consider every patient who walks through the door as a potential adversary. It is a chilling and disconcerting quandary for all of us—being advised to behave like adversaries in the nonadversial, collaborative enterprise of psychotherapy (Kaslow & Schulman, 1987).

Studies of psychotherapists (e.g., Guy et al., 1992; Knapp, VandeCreek, & Phillips, 1993; Wilbert & Fulero, 1988) consistently find them actively worrying about malpractice—both their committing it and patients suing them for it. Between 8 and 23% of clinicians worry about it often—although, again, only 1–2% will actually be charged with malpractice in their careers. In extreme cases, practitioners may develop litigaphobia: the excessive, unreasonable fear of litigation by a patient. Approximately one-quarter of psychologists reported being in a situation—suicide, homicide, child custody evaluations, or fee disputes, for example—that caused them to fear an ethical complaint or a malpractice suit (Knapp et al., 1993).

However, receipt of a malpractice suit or a licensing board complaint is only the beginning of a protracted hellish story. The majority of complaints to a licensing board are ultimately determined to be unfounded, but the investigation process is rough on the psychotherapist nonetheless. A year-long investigation may eventually bring out the truth, but not before the therapist has had to fight for her reputation, defend herself to peers, and survive the mental anguish involved (Kottler, 1986). Most therapists are patently unprepared for the painful consequences and expenses of defending themselves against a complaint (Lewis, 2004). A few therapists even decide to surrender their license and retire rather than face the agony of the investigation.

Coming full circle, we return to Gerry Koocher's nightmarish dream that began this section. The range of stressful patient behaviors seems infinite at times. Our core being is touched again and again—working with terminally ill patients and facing with them their fears of death, or counseling patients with chronic pain caught in a web of hopelessness. Working with physically disabled patients can activate nightmares of our own old age as well as terrors of being confined to a wheelchair. And those conducting family therapy will invariably confront physical violence and emotional abuse in families as well as residual pain from their own family of origin. Independent of the demographics and disorders of the particular client, the core of the therapist as a person is indeed touched again and again.

WORKING CONDITIONS

Ideally, a practitioner's workplace is a holding environment or a safe haven for the psychotherapist perpetually confronted with this laundry list of conflict-ridden patient behaviors. But realistically, the workplace often represents an additional source of stress.

Organizational politics, managed care, excessive paperwork, demanding workloads, and professional conflicts lead the list of complaints of experienced practitioners (e.g., Farber & Heifetz, 1981; Nash, Norcross, & Prochaska, 1984; Norcross, Karg, & Prochaska, 1997). The excruciating slowness of the system, persistent resistance to new ideas, and unrealistic expectations are the key stressors of students entering the helping professions (Corey & Corey, 1989). The cozy setting of psychotherapy—the comfortable armchairs, the warm relationship, intimate engagement—often obscures its hazardous working conditions (Yalom, 2002).

Virtually all healing contexts are dominated by a sense of damage, despair, and disease. And that's only with the patients! Once you add in the bureaucratic nonsense, colleague misbehavior, inadequate resources, onerous paperwork, and assorted organizational and peer problems, one begins to recognize the potential damage of "working conditions" in the helping professions.

To be sure, different contexts make for different patterns of stress. Virtually every study (e.g., Farber & Heifetz, 1982; Hellman & Morrison, 1987; Orlinsky & Rønnestad, 2005; Raquepaw & Miller, 1989; Rupert & Kent, 2007; Snibbe et al., 1989) finds that psychotherapists employed in institutional and HMO settings experience more distress and burnout symptoms than those employed in private practice. Psychotherapists in private practice, on the other hand, find patient behaviors and financial concerns comparatively more stressful.

The major stresses attending independent practice tend to be, in descending order, managed care, time pressures, economic uncertainty, caseload uncertainty, business-related duties, and excessive workload (Nash et al., 1984; Norcross et al., 1997). Recurrent themes distinctive to independent practitioners include frustrations with insurance companies and third-party reimbursers and unrealistic demands for superhuman feats from clients, insurers, and the court system (Nash et al., 1984). The financial instability and risk associated with full or part-time private practice is a huge source of difficulty (Guy, 1987). And in the absence of firm criteria for client success, therapists are left to define their own terms for success, which often prove to be unrealistic or overly idealistic (Raider, 1989).

Even mental health professionals in administrative positions encounter their own varieties of stress from working conditions. Residency directors experience unique pressures and difficulties—having to select residents, struggling to assure that the faculty provide adequate care, contending with bureaucratic hassles, being overloaded with tasks, and warily monitoring residents released to function independently, to name but a few (Yager & Borus, 1990). Clinical supervisors, similarly, must attend to multiple and occasionally conflicting constituencies: student learning, client welfare, program requirements, and so forth.

We extract three evidence-based conclusions from the research on therapist working conditions. One is that each work setting comes equipped with generic stressors as well as its own unique pressures. A second conclusion is that we must guard against overgeneralizing group differences in work settings to individual practitioners; for example, there are many contented practitioners in agencies and many dissatisfied practitioners in private practice. A third conclusion is that we must adopt a more nuanced perspective on the person–environment interaction. It is not the general work setting or environment per se, but the particular characteristics of that setting, such as low autonomy and low support in some agencies, that pose the greatest hazards. We will return to this latter point repeatedly in Chapter 9, "Creating a Flourishing Environment."

THERAPEUTIC RELATIONSHIPS

The therapeutic relationship constitutes both the agony and the ecstasy of our work. It is, at once, the most significant source of pleasure and displeasure in psychotherapy. We alternate between sleepless nights fraught with recollections of hostility and anxiety incurred from characterlogically impaired patients and fleeting moments of realization that we have genuinely assisted a fellow human being (Brady, Norcross, & Guy, 1995).

Among the most widely reported stressors associated with the therapeutic relationship are the responsibility for the patients' lives, the difficulty in working with disturbed patients, and the lack of gratitude from patients (Farber & Heifetz, 1981). The very process of working intimately with human suffering presents the practitioner with psychic discomfort (Goldberg, 1986). If we are not careful, we wind up carrying around the weight and pain of every single patient, as though we were a mama kangaroo.

An empathic relationship with patients will necessarily activate the pain of countertransference. Ever since Freud identified the phenomenon, overidentification and overinvolvement with the patient, manifested through countertransference, have plagued psychotherapists. Countertransference is often invoked when the practitioner recognizes within herself the client's experience and is caught in the dilemma of trying to empathize with the client's feelings while, at the same time, avoid being adversely affected by them (Goldberg, 1986). Countertransference reactions include the arousal of guilt from unresolved personal struggles, inaccurate interpretations of the client's feelings due to therapist projection, feeling blocked and frustrated with a client, and boredom or impatience during treatment.

Which of us has not been repulsed by the actions and attitudes of a child molester, rapist, thief, or murderer? Of course, not all patients stimulate these feelings; only certain clients evoke such stressful reactions. As psychotherapists, we still struggle with distortions, unconscious reactions, unresolved conflicts, misperceptions, and antagonism in relation to particular clients (Kottler, 1986). Each client rubs the therapist a different way, bringing about different reactions.

Clinical interactions are typically characterized by constant emotional arousal (Raider, 1989). This arousal is simultaneously a curative agent for the client and a damaging one for the therapist. Here lies a recurring irony of clinical work: empathy with the client's distress deepening the therapist's pain. The proper therapeutic relationship demands a delicate balance, namely, remaining open to anguished feelings while retaining a modicum of self-preserving distance.

Lastly, fear of psychopathology as a result of intense contact with disordered individuals may cause a psychotherapist, and particularly a trainee, to experience continual fear and intermittent symptoms (Greenfeld, 1985). Constant exposure to conflict is traumatic, even when it is not your own conflict. Constant exposure reactivates our own personal conflicts, or at least poses the fear of reactivating those conflicts. Examining the psychological disorders of others fosters a great deal of morbid self-examination and symptom overidentification. Identifying with the patient's psychopathology while simultaneously striving to maintain the necessary psychological mindedness can pose significant challenges to our own mental health (Doyle, 1987).

INDUSTRIALIZATION OF MENTAL HEALTH

Had we written this chapter in the 1980s or early 1990s, we would have apprised you of the classic stressors confronting the mental health practitioner: demanding patients, organizational politics, emotional exhaustion, and professional isolation. But during the past two decades new and evolving stressors have appeared, namely, increased demands for speed, numbers, and paperwork. The typical practitioner is now threatened with being overwhelmed by the escalating number of patients per day, the 30- to 40-minute sessions, the average of three to eight sessions, the mounting paperwork for diagnoses, treatment plans, and accountability. There is no longer a threat of professional isolation; on the contrary, the real threat is frenetic overinvolvement with patients, colleagues, insurance carriers, and administrators. All this represents a sea change not only in mental health treatment but also in the stressors endured by the terribly human clinician.

The angst and disillusionment practitioners feel toward managed care are almost palpable. Many speak of the "catastrophe that overshadows our profession" and, after careers dedicated to the profession of psychotherapy, find themselves "reduced to numbers in corporate computers" (Graham, 1995, p. 4). The shadow of health care industrialization is looming: many practitioners are losing money, patients, and, perhaps most urgently, autonomy.

Health care has manifested the two cardinal characteristics of any industrial revolution (Cummings, 1986, 1988). First, the producer—in our case, the psychotherapist—is losing control over the services as this control shifts to business interests. Control of psychotherapy is shifting to the payer, with associated shifts in goals and toward limits in reimbursable treatments. Second, practitioners' incomes are decreasing, because industrialization minimizes labor costs. Not surprisingly, income surveys consistently demonstrate that, as a group, psychotherapists are indeed losing income, when adjusted for inflation. Depending on the survey and the methodology, beginning around 1995 doctoral-level psychotherapists averaged 2–5% less net income per year; adjusting for inflation, they lost even more (e.g., *Psychotherapy Finances*, 2004; Rothbaum, Bernstein, Haller, Phelps, & Kohout, 1998).

Managed care plans now cover 80%+ of the Americans who receive their health benefits through their employer. The practice patterns of psychotherapists and the income trends are thus evident—at least for the 75–80% of licensed mental health practitioners who accept some managed care insurance. In a study of 487 psychologists, for instance, the median percentages of managed care patients in psychologists' caseload increased tenfold—from 5 to 50%—over a 4-year period during the mid-1990s (Norcross et al., 1997).

The strain on psychotherapists is immediately linked to managed care—or managed costs and mangled care, if you prefer—but the overarching stress lies in the industrialization of mental health care. Managed care is not a monolithic entity, but most of us know the symptoms of "managing" psychotherapy (Norcross & Knight, 2000):

- Restricting access to treatment (e.g., only "medically necessary" services for Axis I disorders)
- Limiting the amount of psychotherapy (e.g., to 4–10 sessions)
- Using lower-cost providers (e.g., baccalaureate-level therapists)
- Implementing utilization review (e.g., after 3 or 4 sessions)
- Approving primarily short-term, symptom-focused psychotherapies
- Referrals only via the primary care physician gatekeepers
- Restricting patients' freedom of choice in providers and treatments

The restrictions of managed care impact all mental health professionals, but especially independent practitioners. The external constraints, additional paperwork, and lower reimbursement rates are the most highly rated stressors (Rupert & Baird, 2004). In contrast to colleagues with low managed care involvement, practitioners with high managed care involvement worked long hours, received less supervision, saw more clients, experienced more stress, reported more negative client behaviors, and scored higher on emotional exhaustion (Rupert & Baird, 2004). 'Tis a recipe for burnout and diminished self-care.

Fully 80% of 15,918 psychologists responding to a survey (Phelps, Eisman, & Kohout, 1998) reported managed care as having a negative impact (26% high negative, 37% medium negative, and 17% low negative impact). When asked to endorse the top practice concerns from a list of 18, the psychologists most frequently nominated concerns related to managed care: managed care changing clinical practice; income decreased due to managed care fee structure; excess precertification and utilization review requirements of managed care panels; and ethical conflicts raised by managed care. The rhinoceros is in the house, friends, and its name is "managed care."

HAZARDS INHERENT IN THE PERSON OF THE PSYCHOTHERAPIST

Most of the aforementioned hazards "come with the territory." They are part of the world of the psychotherapist. We find ways to minimize their impact, but few of us can avoid them altogether.

At the same time, some practitioners create additional hazards that undermine their satisfaction and well-being over the course of a career.

These are rooted in the therapist's personal history and earlier life experiences, factors that may have led to the vocational choice of psychotherapy and that interact with ongoing life events (Freudenberger, 1990b; Keinan, Almagor, & Ben-Porath, 1989).

Motivations for Becoming a Psychotherapist

Several of the characteristics that attract individuals to a mental health career—commitment to altruism and self-knowledge, for instance—lay the foundation for later disappointments and problems. The source of our success can also be the root of the problem.

It is widely joked that some of the strangest individuals select psychotherapy as a career. Behind this humorous stereotype lies some truth. Many entering the profession are understandably motivated by curiosity about their own personalities. They hope to find solutions to personal problems or some resolution of underlying conflicts (Elliot & Guy, 1993; Goldberg, 1986). If the personal distress motivating this career choice is serious enough, the pressures inherent in conducting psychotherapy will exacerbate emotional problems (Overholser & Fine, 1990). Pursuing a career as a psychotherapist primarily out of a desire to relieve emotional distress is a venture likely to lead to disillusionment.

A related characteristic is a tendency to be drawn to the intimate encounters of psychotherapy out of a desire to combat loneliness. As a group, psychotherapists had relatively few friends before adulthood and tend to be loners (Henry, Sims, & Spray, 1973). The reality of practitioner isolation and artificial intimacy found in the work does little to satisfy interpersonal longings and attachment needs. If anything, the intense encounters with clients may serve to heighten rather than lessen the desire for love and understanding in a person who has yet to find satisfying relationships in her personal life.

Some psychotherapists are motivated to enter the profession in part because it provides the chance to exercise influence or vicariously live through patients. Therapeutic practice offers the temptation to vicariously act out personal fantasies, conflicts, and desires by encouraging clients toward a particular perspective (Bugental, 1964). Psychotherapists indeed want to "make a difference," but this motive can possibly deteriorate into a god-like position of control for a charismatic individual (Guggenbuhl-Craig, 1971). The psychotherapist's power can be considerable, and the resultant sense of self-importance can be intoxicating for those who secretly worry about their own competence as a professional and effectiveness as a person. Arrogance and grandiosity are occupational hazards that can also transfer to the home setting.

Some individuals are drawn to this career due to the unspoken belief that their caring has special curative powers. In a near messianic fashion, they feel compelled to pour out their love on others with the expectation that it will serve as an emotional salve or balm. Such uber-altruism leads them to ignore their own needs—caring for others but not for themselves. It is easy to see how this motivator can lead to a false sense of omnipotence or, on the contrary, an enormous sense of disillusionment when the truth becomes known.

Some clinicians were born into or assigned the role of caretaker at an early age in their families of origin. The resultant career motives can be less than ideal (Dryden & Spurling, 1989; Guy, 1987). Whether assigned or naturally predisposed to the role of "helper," such therapists find little reason to continue if personal growth leads to new interests and roles. Of course, there are likely to be some who have looked to a career in psychotherapy in order to resolve personal needs related to family dysfunction. This motivation is also likely to lose its relevance over time. Systemic changes are likely to be very modest, if they occur at all, and the need to rescue/repair these relationships eventually diminishes as the therapist resolves her conflicts regarding the family of origin.

Intercurrent Life Events

Stressors in the therapist's life outside of the consulting room receive too little attention (Guy, 1987). Life has an uncanny knack of interfering with our plans to create the ideal clinical encounter that reflects only the client's need. In truth, the clinical encounter reflects the combined reality of both the client and therapist.

Life events can cause considerable distress in the therapist's inner world. In several of our studies (e.g., Guy, Poelstra, & Stark, 1989; Norcross & Prochaska, 1986a; Prochaska & Norcross, 1983), between 75 and 82% of psychotherapists reported experiencing a distressing episode within the past 3 years, and more than one-third of these respondents indicated that these personal problems diminished the quality of their patient care. In another study (Pope, Tabachnick, & Keith-Spiegel, 1987), 62% of psychotherapists admitted to working when too distressed to be effective. The most common precipitating events of distressed psychotherapists are disruptions in their own lives—dysfunctional marriages, serious illnesses, and other interpersonal losses—as opposed to client problems (Norcross & Aboyoun, 1994).

Our emotionally taxing profession frequently places stress on the marital or partner relationship (Freudenberger, 1990b). The therapist's psychological mindedness may cause her to respond to a partner in a "therapeutic" manner, leaving the partner feeling estranged and misunderstood. In one survey of therapists' personal problems (Deutsch, 1985), over three-fourths of the respondents reported having experienced relationship difficulties. Another study (Thoreson et al., 1989) found that over 10% of psychologists experienced high levels of distress due to marital or relational dissatisfaction. And several studies (e.g., Wahl et al., 1993) have found correlations between psychotherapist stress and marital dissatisfaction, suggesting that increased work stress is related to decreased marital satisfaction.

Pregnancy is another significant life event that has ramifications for both male and female therapists. The first pregnancy brings profound changes in roles and lifestyles as well as the therapist–patient relationship (Guy, Guy, & Liaboe, 1986). For female therapists, pregnancy is a nonverbal communication to patients, destroying any anonymity (Paluszny & Pozanski, 1971) in that it becomes obvious that the therapist has a personal life that involves sexual activity and family ties (Ashway, 1984). Many pregnant therapists fear being less attentive to patients and becoming increasingly self-absorbed with thoughts and fantasies about the baby (Balsam & Balsam, 1974; Bienen, 1990; Fenster, Phillips, & Rappoport, 1986). Some therapists may feel guilty for becoming pregnant and abandoning their patients to care for the newborn. The growing sense of physical vulnerability, hormonal changes, and fatigue also impact the female therapist's effectiveness (Guy et al., 1986).

Male therapists with pregnant partners may experience many of the same role changes, conflicts, and emotions as the female therapist (Guy et al., 1986). The male therapist may become increasingly preoccupied with concerns for the mother, baby, and his own ability to be an adequate father. Increased financial concerns may heighten his sensitivity to premature terminations and canceled sessions. He may also find himself more reactive to patient disclosures involving pregnancy, parenting, or abortion.

Parenthood supplies an assortment of disruptions in the therapist's relationships with clients. Children become ill, break limbs, and need their parents in emergencies. These realities of parenting increase the complexity of our professional role and necessitate a precarious balancing act to meet the fluid needs of both children and patients (Freudenberger & Robbins, 1979). Common patterns are allowing the therapeutic role to impinge upon family life by overanalyzing and overinterpreting children's behavior (Freudenberger & Kurtz, 1990), pressuring children to appear emotionally healthy at all times (Japenga, 1989), allowing patients to intrude into the home life, and being too tired and emotionally drained to engage in family relationships (Golden & Farber, 1998; Kaslow & Schulman, 1987). In fact, 75% of psychotherapists complain that work issues spill over into their family life (e.g., Farber & Heifetz, 1981; Piercy & Wetchler, 1987). The therapist's family may come to resent the energy and caring that seems more available to patients. Exhorting clients to devote more time and energy to nurturing their own family may take on an empty, even hypocritical, ring to many therapists neglecting their own.

Personal disruptions frequently take the form of loss—divorce and the empty nest being two of dozens of examples. Divorce may precipitate therapists' anxiety over its possible discovery by patients or cause doubts concerning competency since their marriage has failed (Guy, 1987). Children "moving out" may precipitate feelings of abandonment, despair, and depletion. Therapists who experience these losses may find terminations with their patients especially difficult (Kaslow & Schulman, 1987). In a study of terminations, we found that therapists significantly affected by the recent departure of children from their home reported a desire for more gradual terminations with their clients (Guy et al., 1993). Similarly, the study found that those therapists substantially affected by divorce were more likely to maintain social contact with clients after termination. Therapeutic relationships may thus be (mis)used to compensate for the losses in therapists' personal lives.

Dissatisfaction with their personal life is the leading precipitant of psychotherapists' engaging in a sexual relationship with a patient. Feeling lonely or alienated, moving through a divorce or a dying parent, enduring relationship crises, and financial concerns lead the list (Lamb, Catanzaro, & Moorman, 2003). Some 2–6% of psychologists (overwhelmingly male) report sexual relationships with clients (during or after treatment), which is prohibited by ethical codes (Lamb et al., 2003). These sexual boundary violations are tied directly to both intercurrent life events and past personal vulnerabilities.

As a psychotherapist ages into late adulthood, it becomes increasingly difficult to keep personal concerns from influencing professional practice. The death of loved ones, the physical and mental effects of aging, and personal illnesses all exacerbate the depletion of the therapist's abilities (King, 1983). Aging or ailing psychotherapists often experience anxiety as they confront, perhaps for the first time, the reality of their own mortality (Guy & Souder, 1986a, 1986b). Some therapists feel guilty about becoming ill and having to temporarily "abandon" their patients (Schwartz, 1987); others experiencing vulnerability and helplessness increase their desire to be cared for by their clients. This sense of weakness can be quite disturbing to the therapist who typically perceives herself to be strong and competent (Dewald, 1982).

BURNOUT

In the opening chapter, we argued that striving to prevent burnout is a more pathological and less effective strategy than cultivating self-care. Nonetheless, no chapter on the occupational hazards of psychotherapists would be complete without a few paragraphs on burnout.

Burnout has been defined in a variety of ways (e.g., Freudenberger & Richelson, 1980; Perlman & Hartman, 1982; Guy, 1987), but it always links directly to emotional depletion. We endorse the definition of burnout as "physical and emotional exhaustion, involving the development of negative self-concept, negative job attitudes, and loss of concern and feelings for clients" (Pines & Maslach, 1978, p. 233). Thus, when the emotional drain from work-related factors is so great that it hinders personal and professional functioning, the therapist is likely suffering from burnout.

Solid research indicates that approximately 2–6% of psychotherapists are experiencing burnout at any one time (Farber, 1990; Farber & Norcross, 2005). However, 32% of the therapists experience symptoms of burnout and depression to a degree serious enough to interfere with their work, and a similar 26% believe their colleagues suffer from symptoms related to burnout and depression (Wood, Klein, Cross, Lammers, & Elliot, 1985). Thus, while the vast majority of psychotherapists are emotionally "good enough" at any given time, periodic "brownouts" and instances of clinical burnout are prevalent.

There is no need here for an extensive summary of the mounting literature on psychotherapist burnout; however, we would like to punctuate three critical points. First, one should fully appreciate the interactive effects of occupational stress and psychotherapist personality. It is not simply the stressful environment nor solely the vulnerable person, but truly the interaction between the environment and person. The upshot: each psychotherapist must sort through the unique array of environmental work stressors that confront her and then address the iterative, idiosyncratic impacts on her own world. For example, the two of us experience physical isolation very differently. It troubles one of us not an iota, the other quite a bit. Surely this says something important about our personality and predispositions. Surely, too, this says we must individually tailor our self-care to these personality predispositions.

A second critical point: burnout is not a unitary or global disorder; there are distinct subtypes of burnout with attendant different self-care strategies. Several subtypes have been empirically delineated (Farber, 1998): wearout or brownout, in which a practitioner essentially gives up or performs in a perfunctory manner when confronted with too much stress and too little gratification; classic or frenetic burnout, in which the practitioner works increasingly hard to the point of exhaustion in pursuit of sufficient gratification to match the extent of stress experienced; and underchallenged burnout, in which a practitioner is not faced with work overload but rather with monotonous and unstimulating work that fails to provide sufficient rewards. Each type requires a different self-care solution.

Our third and final critical point is that the probability of burnout is reliably associated with several identifiable risk factors (Guy, 1987). Here is a brief summary of a lengthy literature. Psychotherapist characteristics: loners who are idealistic, dedicated, and service-oriented; high desire for recognition and positive feedback; married women with children (Gadzella, Ginther, Tomcala, & Bryant, 1991; Freudenberger & Robbins, 1979). Patient characteristics: suicidal, violent, hostile, aggressive, and excessively demanding patients; frequent premature terminations; seeing the same kind of client hour after hour. Job requirements: role ambiguity, role conflict, role overload, and role inconsequentiality (Farber, 1983b, 1983c). Working conditions: high job stress, inadequate supervisor support, inadequate organizational resources, and large number of hours worked (Poulin & Walter, 1993a, 1993b).

RESPONDING TO THE HAZARDS

Lions, and tigers, and bears! Oh my! What a staggering list of hazards and burdens. Are we trying to drive you out of the profession and into real estate sales? Not hardly. So, here are the tradeoffs, and here are the ultimate purposes of this chapter.

Recognition

Our selves are our therapeutic tools. To put our problem in a nutshell (Lasky, 2005): Is there any kind of work in this world where the tools never get dull, chipped, or broken?

We began this chapter by saying it out loud and will do so again: Psychotherapy is often a grueling and demanding calling. Be aware of the occupational hazards inherent in the work and those unique to your work setting and personal vulnerabilities. Establish realistic expectations. Expect to feel overwhelmed and drained at times. Beware of what pushes your button, rings your bell, and activates your neuroses.

When recognizing the stresses you encounter as a psychotherapist, keep in mind that similar kinds of pressure are experienced by virtually all of your colleagues. Confidentiality, isolation, shame, and a host of additional considerations lead us to overpersonalize our own sources of stress when in reality they are part and parcel of the "common world" of psychotherapy. Disconfirming our individual feelings of unique wretchedness and affirming the universality of stresses are in and of themselves therapeutic.

Although we psychotherapists face the same trials and tribulations, we are hesitant to admit it publicly. The autobiographical accounts of experienced psychotherapists (e.g., Burton, 1972; Dryden & Spurling,

1989; Goldfried, 2001) make it painfully clear that they have experienced many of the same personal tragedies, failures, and stressors as the rest of us. Despite our secret fantasy that prominent therapists may have discovered a way to inoculate themselves against the ravages of distress, experience proves otherwise. In the words of Freud (1905/1933): "No one who, like me, conjures up the most evil of those half-tamed demons that inhabit the human breast, and seeks to wrestle with them, can expect to come through the struggle unscathed."

Acceptance

Appreciating the universality of these hazards and accepting some of their inevitable distress contribute to the creation of corrective actions. Speaking of corrective actions: let us accept from the outset that our positions exact considerable demands for high-quality work. Acceptance is a crucial mindset, as our cognitive-behavioral colleagues have learned in terms of treatment methods and our psychoanalytic colleagues have informed us in terms of a tragic view of human nature. Acceptance is an active process, not a passive resignation.

Here's how we personally think about it: Clinicians already have two strikes against them. Freud, as you will recall, christened psychotherapy an impossible profession. But it was only one of three that he identified; the others were education and politics or governing (depending on the translation). Thus, clinicians are daily practicing two of the impossible professions—psychotherapy and politics or government—depending on your involvement in agency politics, professional organizations, and administrative responsibilities. That's our acceptance strategy—we are involved in highly gratifying but impossible pursuits, and keeping our nose above the waterline is doing well under the circumstances.

Self-Empathy

Another place to begin is to *Start Where You Are*, the title of a book by the Buddhist nun Pema Chodron (1994). "Our first step is to develop compassion for our own wounds. . . . It is unconditional compassion for us that leads naturally to unconditional compassion for others. If we are willing to stand fully in our own shoes and never give up on ourselves, then we will be able to put ourselves in the shoes of others and never give up on them" (p. x).

Team Approach

In appreciating the universality of occupational hazards and in cultivating self-empathy, you will probably discover that high-stress clinical situations require a team approach. The death of a child, severe PTSD, and suicidal borderline pathology, for instance, require multiple professionals working together (e.g., Kazak & Noll, 2004; Linehan, 1993). It is too much for a single clinician; it is inhumane for one person to go it alone. A team can better share the burden, process the pain, manage countertransference, and support one another.

Your team comes in many guises. The team may be an interdisciplinary cadre working directly with you on a particular case. The team may be supervisors, peers, and personal therapists. Your team may be researchers publishing on the disorder or dilemma you are confronting, your profession advancing your cause for equitable reimbursement for your services, or colleagues (like us) offering workshops and books on replenishing yourself. We devote several later chapters to self-care via nurturing professional and personal relationships, but did want to highlight here that you need not be alone and need not go it alone clinically.

Tailor Self-Care to the Individual

In this chapter, we have followed the conventional typology of therapist stressors in terms of sources—physical and emotional isolation, patient behaviors, working conditions, therapeutic relationships, and so on. Another scheme is to conceptualize therapists' practice difficulties in terms of three types:

1. *Transient* difficulties based on competency deficits; we literally do not know what to do or how to do something.
2. *Paradigmatic* difficulties based on therapists' enduring personality characteristics.
3. *Situational* difficulties based on features of particular patients and circumstances (Schroder & Davis, 2004).

Here's the payoff of this typology: different types of difficulties call for differential responses. Transient difficulties call for improved knowledge, training, and wider experiences; situational difficulties require tolerance, support, and acceptance; and paradigmatic difficulties call for enhanced self-awareness and countertransference measures.

To disentangle the three types, ask yourself questions: Have you come across such a difficulty outside of the practice setting? With other patients? How are other therapists experiencing the situation? Would training and skill enhancement solve the problem? And so on (Schroder & Davis, 2004).

As you assess your own difficulties, attend to the types you experience and then develop a corresponding self-care plan. Some difficulties call for peer acceptance and colleague support ("That damn supervisor!"

"Can't understand this new form"), some call for training ("I need to learn more about treating trauma"), and still others for supervision or personal therapy ("It's happening with another patient, just as it does in my personal life"). Different folks need different self-care strokes.

Tradeoffs and Balance

The hazards of psychotherapeutic practice must be reconciled and balanced with its privileges. Our work's frustrations are only half the story. In the lyrics of Jackson Browne's (1974) song, "Fountain of sorrow, fountain of light."

Our esteemed colleague, Jim Bugental (1978, pp. 149–150), put the tradeoffs beautifully. His 40+ years of practicing psychotherapy have profoundly changed him:

> My life as a psychotherapist has been . . . the source of anguish, pain, and anxiety—sometimes in the work itself, but more frequently within myself and with those important in my life. Similarly that work and those relationships have directly and indirectly brought to me and those in my life joy, excitement, and a sense of participation in truly vital experiences.

As with most meaningful endeavors, a career as a psychotherapist is a mixed bag of benefits and liabilities. Few careers offer the rewards experienced by the dedicated clinician, as we described in Chapter 2. Yet, most psychotherapists discover that encounters with distressed individuals and repeated confrontations with the painful aspects of human existence can undermine vitality and optimism.

The therapist who denies that clinical work is grueling and demanding is, in Thorne's (1988) view, mendacious, deluded, or incompetent. We concur wholeheartedly, but would add that the therapist who claims not to have personally benefited from this grueling and demanding work is also likely to be mendacious, deluded, or incompetent. Without trivializing the enormous strains associated with this impossible profession, we would conclude that most of us feel enriched, nourished, and privileged in conducting clinical work.

The Long Perspective

To avoid the impression that psychotherapy is indeed an impossible profession, it's important to place the content of this chapter in perspective. Most psychotherapists enjoy long, successful careers during which time they experience only a relative few of the hazards we have discussed. When they do encounter these challenges, they are typically able to overcome them. This reflects the quality of their personal awareness, support network, and resilience. It also reminds us that practically all of us use several of the self-care strategies described throughout this book.

If you—like us—have recognized ways in which you have been harmed by the practice of psychotherapy, please be concerned but not alarmed. The liabilities associated with clinical practice can be reduced by a variety of concrete and creative measures. The remainder of this book specifically addresses skillful self-care mindsets and methods that have emerged from the recognition of occupational hazards.

Our genuine hope is that the material contained in this chapter, although temporarily disconcerting, will assist you in summoning the conceptual and experiential tools required for a long, satisfying career as a mental health professional. In the remainder of this volume, our aim is to share what our colleagues, experience, and research have taught us about overcoming the distress of conducting psychotherapy.

SELF-CARE CHECKLIST

✓ Repeat the mantra "Psychotherapy is often a grueling and demanding calling" frequently in order to establish realistic expectations.

✓ Affirm the universality of occupational hazards by sharing your stressors and distress with trusted colleagues.

✓ Identify the impact of clinical practice on you and your loved ones. All accounts indicate that clinical practice exacts a negative toll on the practitioner, particularly in the form of problematic anxiety, moderate depression, and emotional underinvolvement with family members.

✓ Consider the amount of physical isolation you experience each day. What steps can you take to create more opportunities for contact with other clinicians?

✓ Create variety in your day, such as intermingling psychotherapy sessions with supervision, consultations, study breaks, a trip to the gym, and so on.

✓ Invite family and friends to point out when you become too interpretive and "objective" when it would be healthier to be spontaneous and genuine.

✓ Know the actuarial data about the probability of a malpractice lawsuit or licensing complaint and thoughtfully consider the high-risk aspects of your practice (e.g., your involvement with borderline and narcissistic personality disorders, suicidal and violent patients, "recovered memory" cases, contested divorce cases).

✓ Calculate the possibility of patient violence in your office and take steps to enhance your personal safety accordingly.

✓ Take coach John Wooden's advice and refuse to believe either your most idealizing or your most demeaning client—you are neither God nor the devil.

✓ Limit your exposure to traumatic images outside the therapy room by choosing movies, literature, and other entertainment carefully.

✓ Reevaluate your involvement with managed care, particularly its possible contribution to your experience of depletion and burnout. How might you restore some control in your work to enhance your sense of autonomy?

✓ Adopt a team approach in dealing with high-stress clinical situations; distribute the burden and lighten the individual load.

✓ Beware of inadvertent domestic violations of patient confidentiality, and limit the amount of client material you share with your significant others.

✓ Consider how you have managed the delicate balance between empathic connection and self-preserving distance in your clinical work. When you find yourself on one end of the pendulum, pursue balance.

✓ Reflect on the number of clients that you've said good-bye to over the years. What has been the cumulative impact of these terminations?

✓ Address your own limitations and needs in an open manner instead of playing competitive therapist games.

✓ Periodically reevaluate why you became a psychotherapist and why you continue to practice. Look for ways to work through those unhealthy motivations.

✓ Proactively discuss your professional and parental commitments within significant relationships.

✓ Accept some spillover from your professional life into your personal life as an inevitable cost of being human.

✓ Discuss with your spouse/partner the topics covered in this chapter. How does he or she perceive their impact on your relationship?

✓ Learn how to handle distracting intercurrent life events. Perhaps consult with a trusted and more experienced colleague.

✓ Implement proactive steps to reduce the low but real possibility of burnout.

✓ "Start where you are": cultivate self-empathy regarding occupational hazards so that you can develop empathy for others.

✓ Tailor your self-care to your personality and context by disentangling transient, paradigmatic, and situational difficulties in your practice; each requires a different self-care plan.

✓ Reconcile and balance the hazards of psychotherapeutic practice with its rewards—"fountain of sorrow, fountain of light."

✓ Adopt the long perspective as a healing practitioner; most psychotherapists enjoy lengthy successful careers and would elect to do it again.

RECOMMENDED READING

Dryden, W. (Ed.). (1995). *The stresses of counselling in action.* London: Sage. *www.friedsocialworker.com* (website)

Freudenberger, H. J., & Richelson, G. (1980). *Burn out: How to beat the high cost of success.* New York: Bantam.

Schaufeli, W. B., Maslach, C., & Marek, T. (Eds.). (1993). *Professional burnout: Recent developments in theory and research.* Washington, DC: Taylor & Francis.

Sussman, M. B. (Ed.). (1995). *A perilous calling: The hazards of psychotherapy practice.* New York: Wiley.

CHAPTER 4

Minding the Body

Psychotherapists are so intent and focused on sophisticated self-care methods that we frequently overlook the biobehavioral basics of self-care: adequate sleep, rest, nutrition, exercise, and human contact. Do you subsist during the practice day, as did one of us for years, on diet soda and pretzels between appointments? How many hours of sleep do you need—versus what you typically get? Do you sit all day, major muscles stiffening, while your facial muscles work overtime expressing emotions? Let's not neglect the fundamentals of self-care.

As authors, we half apologize for reminding a sophisticated audience of these basic needs. Yet, the biology is elemental and demanding. The body in psychotherapy has become marginalized; many therapists have historically practiced from the head up. We need to take our bodily reactions more seriously, as the body constitutes the fountainhead of human experience. As Freud repeatedly reminded us, being a psychotherapist does not make us any less human.

In this brief but necessary chapter, we mind the body of the psychotherapist: sleep, bodily rest, nutrition, exercise, and human contact (including sexual gratification). These, quite literally, embody our energy and sense of engagement.

SLEEP

In our interviews with master practitioners, a recurrent self-care theme is obtaining ample sleep—a simple but powerful solution to occupational distress. Said one: "I have really made an effort, though not always a successful one, to get 8 hours of sleep a night. It makes a huge difference."

Our watchword as psychotherapists should be *"Mens sana in corpore sano"* (A healthy mind in a healthy body). It's extremely shortsighted to see sleep as an obstacle to productivity. A nightly investment in sufficient rest leads to greater resilience and accomplishment.

The research literature attests to the value of maintaining a standard sleep window to secure sufficient sleep. Some call this sleep hygiene and others label it sleep stimulus control, but whatever name is used, many meta-analyses support its efficacy for obtaining sleep and treating insomnia (Morin et al., 1999; Smith et al., 2002). Those same meta-analyses further demonstrate that sleep stimulus control typically results in a shorter sleep latency (the amount of time needed to fall asleep) and in fewer negative side effects and addictive consequences than sleep medications.

Stimulus control instructions mesh well with our emphasis in this book on the superior self-care effectiveness of harnessing the power of both the person and the environment. Consider adopting the following sleep rules or instructions (Bootzin, 2005): Lie down intending to go to sleep only when you are sleepy. (This rule strengthens the bed and bedroom as behavioral cues for sleep.) Do not use the bed for anything except sleep; do not read, watch television, or eat in bed. (This rule weakens the association of the bed with activities that might interfere with sleep.) If you find yourself unable to fall asleep, get up and go into another room. (This rule dissociates the bed from the frustration and arousal of not being able to sleep.) Stay up as long as you wish and then return to the bedroom to sleep. Get out of bed if you do not fall asleep within 10–15 minutes. (The goal is to associate the bed with falling asleep quickly.) Do this as often as necessary throughout the night. Set your alarm and get up at the same time every morning irrespective of how much sleep you got during the night. (This rule helps the body to acquire a consistent sleep rhythm). Do not nap during the day (for those suffering from sleep disturbance).

One of us (JCN) has been impressed in his own life with the results of rising with the sun and sleeping with the stars, 10:00 P.M. to 6:00 A.M. It is a highly natural—in tune with nature—sleep pattern. It also gets us to the office early for concentrated stress-free work.

Let's start comprehensive self-care by tending to your sleep, thereby recharging your battery. A body in motion deserves predictable rest.

BODILY REST

The lyrics of Jackson Browne's song, "Running on Empty," warn us that running on empty, without rest or restoration, means pushing harder and enduring more pressure. Running on empty frequently means "running blind" and "running behind."

Psychotherapy consists of two or more physical presences in the consulting room. Interviews with experienced psychotherapists reveal that they suffer physically in a number of ways from the craft (Shaw, 2004). When we are empathic, we respond physically to patients, such as an anorexic or bulimic patient talking about vomiting and diarrhea. We vicariously feel anxiety as patients describe a panic attack or physical abuse. The body is a receiver.

The stress associated with conducting psychotherapy is often manifested in muscle tension, particularly in the jaw, neck, and back. As a result, many of us find massage to be an effective and pleasurable method of treating muscle discomfort. Facial massages are natural antidotes to experiencing and expressing strong emotions through the major face muscles. Massage not only helps muscles relax but also clears away waste products and the assorted pain that comes with tight muscles. Physiologically, it stimulates blood flow, improves muscle tone, and enhances the immune function (Field, 1998). Psychologically, a course of massage therapy reduces anxiety and depression almost as much as psychotherapy, according to a meta-analysis of 37 studies (Moyer, Rounds, & Hannum, 2004).

Our muscles stiffen when we sit for such long hours. In the office, we have learned to take short walks between sessions, even if only within the office or to the bathroom, and to give ourselves facial massages to ease the tension in the jaw. Outside the office, we have learned to schedule full-body hour-long massages.

Massage offers a recuperative rest from the turbulence of stress (Cady & Jones, 1997; Field, 1998). As stated by one master therapist: "I go to a professional massage therapist once a month or more. It helps keep me in touch with my body. It also reverses the roles; I am in the position of receiving rather than giving the care." Another master clinician used massage in a creative and specific manner:

> "I was doing marital therapy with a couple, and they were really struggling with some issues that were difficult for me to be emotionally present to. What I did during the course of seeing them in therapy was set up a weekly session of massage for myself. I experimented with having my massage session before seeing the couple versus after seeing the couple. Although it felt good afterward, it seemed to be more helpful ahead of time. It helped me be centered and balanced and emotionally present in terms of what they were experiencing and my being moderator and counselor."

Different massage techniques are readily available from professionals in virtually all localities: deep muscle, Swedish, hot stone, acupressure, Rolfing, and more. Taking a class or receiving individual treatments can be most useful, both for immediate stress reduction and for ongoing body self-care. We urge you to try it if you haven't already. It is simply invaluable.

During sessions in the office, try to keep your body straight and sit erect. Some therapists appear to flop around or remain off-kilter. The therapist's physical posture is a crucial indicator. Sitting with a good posture throughout the session helps you give clients your full attention and preserves your energy. Be balanced and flexible, always gravitating to your center (Rosenbaum, 1999).

Move your body often to counteract the sedentary nature of your workday. Go for brief walks between appointments or during lunch. Learn to massage your own feet between sessions. Make sure you stretch your shoulders, neck, and legs now and then. Avoid a motionless sitting position that reduces your circulation and energy. In sum, give your body a rest between the relentlessly emotional but sedentary sessions.

NUTRITION AND HYDRATION

In one of our first workshops on self-care, we quizzed the participants privately and anonymously about their nutrition during the workday. Only a quarter of psychotherapists thought their nutritional intake was healthy and adequate; three-quarters thought it was unhealthy, inadequate, or both. Since that inauspicious discovery, we always take a few moments to address nutrition and hydration.

Up until the past 10 years, our own performance in this domain of biobehavioral self-care was dismal. We subsisted throughout the day on coffee, sodas, and quick finger foods, only to become ravished and eat one humungous, unhealthy meal at 9 P.M. We have become more mindful of our nutrition of late—perhaps because we are heeding our own advice, perhaps because we are in middle age, or perhaps because our caring spouses are determined to improve us. (Our money is on the latter.)

One of our psychotherapy patients was a registered dietician who helpfully suggested that we monitor our fluid intake during the workday. After thanking her for the recommendation and commenting on her reenactment of devoting more time to others than to herself (her presenting problem for treatment!), we gratefully did so. We were consuming about 60% of the recommended daily intake of 3 liters (13 cups) for men (2.2 liters for women; Institute of Medicine, 2006). Losing just 2% of your body's water will result in your feeling tired and weak. You might want to monitor your own hydration for a few clinical days.

The self-care imperative is to eat balanced nutritious meals and to hydrate oneself adequately during the day. Following a self-care workshop, one of our participants wrote: "I've begun by addressing some basic thing and have made a commitment to myself to do something not spectacular but something no matter how small but that builds on my daily self-care. Today it was getting breakfast, listening to relaxing music, and massaging my feet. And so it begins." Exactly so.

EXERCISE

Surveys involving thousands of psychotherapists discover that 71–78% engage in regular physical exercise (Barrow, English, & Pinkerton, 1987; Mahoney, 1997; Sherman & Thelen, 1998). Jogging, walking, workouts, tennis, racquetball, swimming, and bicycling lead the list of favored activities (Barrow et al., 1987). Here are 10 verbatim testimonials from our master clinicians and workshop participants:

- "If I start slowing down or getting a little tired, I go to the gym and I feel better. I go to the gym twice a week, and I do the stationary bicycle for half-an-hour and weights for half-an-hour. That does something that allows me to cope with therapy and the rest of my work much better."
- "Twice a week I go to the YMCA. I join an hour of aerobics and then walking two hours on the track. While I'm walking I think about whatever I want to think about. That helps me get things out of my system."
- "One of the healthy escapes that I use regularly is exercise. I usually swim three times a week at a local club. This allows me to have a complete change of scene from psychotherapy."
- "I play handball four times a week. I spend all day sitting in the office, and handball is a very vigorous game that makes up for the sitting. There is also a social aspect to it. I have been playing with the same people for many years. We are good friends, and we spend. time in the locker room, between games, and after the games to talk and chat about life. They are part of my social support system as well as providing exercise."
- "My most creative ideas often come to me while I am running through the streets on a late afternoon or early morning run. It is an excellent way for me to relieve stress and spend some time outdoors. If I didn't run, I would be crazy by now."
- "Exercise is very good physiologically for stress. It calms me down, and I often have the feeling of literally working off the stress of the day. I do tai chi, which is a type of moving meditation. It is physically demanding, so I get the physiological benefits of exercise. I also get the psychological benefits of meditation. I do this daily."
- "I do three types of exercising: stretching, weight training, and aerobics. I do this at least four times a week. It certainly helps me feel better and clears my mind somewhat."

- "I have made a commitment to exercising several times a week and am actually doing so, blocking out an extended lunch or using time in the morning, and not arriving in my office until 9 A.M. rather than the customary 8 A.M. This has made a tremendous difference."
- "I walk with my patients during some of the therapy sessions. I walk in the office while conducting sessions with adults, and during my sessions with children or adolescents we walk outside. During our walks to nearby stores we talk the entire way. This, both walking inside and outside, helps relieve some of the tension in myself and the patient, and it allows us to talk freer."

A tenth and final illustration comes from Jeffrey Kottler (1986, pp. 138–139) in his book *On Being a Therapist*. Here is his personal testimony on the salubrious effects of exercise:

When I ride my bike the wind washes me clean. Everything I have soaked in during the previous days oozes out through my pores, all the complaints and pain and pressure. I feel only the pain in my legs and lungs as I climb up a hill pumping furiously. And then I coast down as fast as I can, never knowing what is around the next turn. For an hour or two I am no longer a receptacle for other people to dump their suffering. Nobody catches me on my bike. There is no chance to think or I will miss a pothole in the road. And it takes too much concentration watching for traffic, pacing my rhythm, switching gears, working on technique, saving my strength, breathing slow to consider anything outside my body. After a ride through the country, I feel ready again to face my clients, my past, and my uncertain future.

Associations between exercise and well-being have been documented repeatedly for decades. Such exercise most positively impacts the therapist's physical stamina, emotional mood, and mental stamina. The affective beneficence of exercise in psychotherapists converges, of course, with the empirical research attesting to the link between exercise and decreases in depression, anxiety, and body hatred (Hays, 1995). A meta-analysis (Stathopoulou et al., 2006) of 11 treatment outcome studies demonstrates large effects for the efficacy of exercise. We suspect exercise may be even a more powerful benefit for psychotherapists—whose jobs are typically highly verbal, sedentary, and nonphysical—than for people generally.

A cautionary word about exercise for the idealistic, perfectionistic practitioner (that's 94.3% of us): please keep your exercise expectations realistic. Heed the sage words of one of our master practitioners: "While my exercise is modest (20–25 minutes of Nordic Track or stationary bike with sit-ups) every other day, I am realistic that I will be more likely to succeed at this level rather than if I set myself impossible goals. Since I am always encouraging my clients to assess both their confidence and their competence when they set goals, I am trying to take my own advice."

HUMAN CONTACT

Psychologist Harry Harlow (1958) was amongst the first, and inarguably the most memorable, to experimentally demonstrate the inborn need for human contact that clinicians have witnessed for centuries. You may recall that Harlow took infant monkeys away from their biological mothers and gave them instead to two artificial, surrogate mothers, one made of wire and one made of cloth. The wire mother was outfitted with a bottle to feed the baby monkey. But the babies rarely stayed with the wire mother longer than it took to get the necessary food. Babies strongly preferred cuddling with the softer cloth mother, especially when they were frightened, even though it/she did not offer milk.

Such contact comfort is of overwhelming importance in the development of affectional response. Certainly we cannot live by milk alone. We all need contact comfort, a little cuddling.

Some clinicians keep a favorite pillow or afghan nearby during sessions, to hold or touch. Others allow for time for phone calls to close friends and family members in the midst of a busy day. One master clinician schedules a weekly lunch with his spouse and small children, providing an opportunity for physical affection and meaningful contact, between psychotherapy clients.

Of course, the need for contact comfort can be partially satisfied in sexual relationships. Saul Bellow's *Herzog* (1964, p. 166) goes so far as to argue that "the erotic must be admitted to its rightful place, at last, in an emancipated society which understands the relation of sexual repression to sickness, war, property, money, totalitarianism. Why, to get laid is actually socially constructive and useful, an act of citizenship." We would not go that far, but Herzog vividly makes the case for sexual gratification.

The next chapter (Chapter 5) is devoted in its entirety to nurturing relationships for psychotherapists. Our intent here is to collegially remind us all of the biological need for contact comfort and sexual gratification.

IN CLOSING

Psychotherapists, being more human than otherwise, are subject to the same biological needs and amenable to the same physical releases as other humans. In this chapter, we hope to remind you to reconnect to the body, that thing below your neck, in your self-care.

All health care practitioners assuredly know the preceding material and routinely encourage their patients to mind their bodies. But if there is a first-place, blue-ribbon award for the disconnect between psychotherapists' practices with patients and those same psychotherapists' practices with themselves, then it is certainly in the realm of satisfying one's biological needs.

We trust that this chapter has neither belabored the obvious nor insulted your intelligence. Although we have been intentionally brief, let not the chapter's brevity be misconstrued. Sleep, bodily rest, nutrition, exercise, and human contact are indispensable to well-functioning psychotherapists. Get real, get basic, get bodily self-care.

SELF-CARE CHECKLIST

✓ Mind your body as part of your self-care; do not become preoccupied with sophisticated self-care methods at the expense of your biobehavioral basics.

✓ Track the quality and length of your sleep. How many hours of sleep are you averaging each night, compared to what your body needs?

✓ Take your own advice: exercise regularly.

✓ Schedule minibreaks between sessions to self-massage your face, neck, and leg muscles; perhaps schedule regular massages to nourish yourself and relieve muscle tension.

✓ Stretch your muscles and reconnect to your body as antidotes to the sedentary nature of psychotherapy.

✓ Get moving during your workday: go for walks between sessions or during meals and avoid motionless sitting positions that reduce circulation and energy.

✓ Secure sufficient hydration during the day.

✓ Eat balanced, nutritious meals before, during, and after work; avoid the empty calories of comfort foods.

✓ Monitor your use of substances. Are you self-medicating with alcohol, tobacco, drugs, or food?

✓ Arrange for contact comfort and sexual gratification away from the office; it's your responsibility to meet your physical needs.

RECOMMENDED READING

Dement, W. C., & Vaughan, C. (2000). *The promise of sleep.* New York: Dell.

Hays, K. F. (1995). Psychotherapy and exercise behavior change. *Psychotherapy Bulletin, 30*(3), 29–35.

Scott, C. D., & Hawk, J. (Eds.). (1986). *Heal thyself: The health of health care professionals.* New York: Brunner/Mazel.

CHAPTER 5

Nurturing Relationships

In Flannery O'Connor's short story "The Lame Shall Enter First," a psychologist appropriately named Sheppard is dedicated to reforming troubled boys. But the story ends with the devastating realization that, in trying to "save" a particularly hardened boy, Sheppard has neglected his own son and his own soul. "He had stuffed his own emptiness with good works like a glutton," as O'Connor described it. The call to care for others may be taken to overzealous proportions—and with dire consequences (O'Donnell, 1995).

We need to take care while giving care; we need to nurture ourselves while we are nurturing others.

As psychotherapists, we work in a world of intimate relationships. The intense emotions experienced during these encounters seep into our private lives and relationships. As we discussed in Chapter 3, the isolation, introspection, and restraint characteristic of the healer role can reduce our spontaneity, vitality, and spirit. A clinician may notice in herself a growing awkwardness with casual conversation or a tendency to be withdrawn or quiet at parties (Freudenberger, 1990a).

Insofar as intimate treatment relationships can deplete our inner resources, restoration of our resources can also occur within the context of meaningful relationships. Psychotherapists as a group have been described in classic research as independent, socially withdrawn individuals who spend considerable time alone (Henry et al., 1973). Therapists often have the image of a "loner" who restores inner resources by withdrawing into a cocoon of isolation and peace. Indeed, one of our master clinicians described just such a pattern in herself: "After working closely with clients all week, I really look forward to spending time by myself during the weekend. I don't really want to talk to anyone. I'd rather go off alone to hike or bike. Physical recreation, by myself, raises my spirits and gives me back my energy for the next week of appointments."

Despite the occasional need for psychotherapists to recharge their batteries through time spent alone, the clinical and research consensus is that we are best able to restore inner strength and regain emotional balance in the context of meaningful relationships (Medeiros & Prochaska, 1988). In fact, our survey of master therapists for this book found that they relied most heavily on nurturing relationships. As one master clinician put it simply: "I really rely on my most important relationships for personal encouragement. My friends and family give me the love and support I need for dealing with patients all day long."

Nurturing relationships reliably emerge as effective self-care in the psychotherapist research (Norcross & Aboyoun, 1994). In several of our studies, mental health professionals consistently report greater use of helping relationships than educated laypersons in dealing with their own distress. In related studies, increased use of helping relationships correlates positively with psychotherapist well-being—just as use of social support typically does with laypersons (e.g., Pearson, 1986). Expectedly, psychotherapists find helping relationships to be both satisfying and efficacious for themselves.

Of course, psychotherapists find nurturance from their relationships in a multitude of ways. In this chapter, we review advice and examples from a number of these, both in the office (e.g., colleagues, staff, supervisors, sometimes patients) as well as outside the office (e.g., friends, family, consultants).

NURTURING RELATIONSHIPS AT THE OFFICE

The clinical world is frequently populated with individuals capable of providing support, concern, and assistance. Psychotherapists find that they can be replenished by encounters with a variety of people during the workday who give to them the very same expressions of support that they regularly give to clients. This is not to imply that the psychotherapist's role entails an equal share of nurturance for herself; we rarely receive the same amount of caring that we give at the office. Nonetheless, that nurturing moments can come for the therapist within the context of clinical work is indeed a welcomed realization.

Clinical Colleagues

Clinical colleagues are an important means by which to replenish our emotional reserves (Gram, 1992; Lewis, Greenburg, & Hatch, 1988; Menninger, 1991). Because they understand the world in which psychotherapy operates, they are able to appreciate the feelings, reactions, and concerns of fellow psychotherapists. By sharing their perspectives on treatment methods, diagnostic questions, ethical dilemmas, and practice challenges, they become partners who support and advise. This can be quite encouraging and reassuring to the practitioner, who otherwise feels alone with the challenges inherent in her work. Within the defined limits of confidentiality and ethical practice, other psychotherapists are a valuable self-care source.

Most of our master clinicians found it helpful to discuss clinical problems and difficult clients with colleagues as a means of lessening the distress of practicing psychotherapy. Some found it helpful to limit contacts with colleagues to informal encounters in the hallway or casual conversations over lunch. One master clinician described his experiences as follows:

> "I use casual conversations with colleagues to cathart and ventilate my frustrations. It's comforting when one of them says, 'Gee, I am glad to see that that happens to you also and not just to me.' Just the fact that I've shared my complaints makes me feel better . . . simply being able to get if off my chest. It's also helpful to get direction and guidance from colleagues. I walk away fortified by their input."

The authors (Coster & Schwebel, 1997, p. 10) of a study on well-functioning psychologists unambiguously conclude their study by stating, "If you do not have a close, cooperative, trusting relationship with one or more colleagues, we advise you to establish one. Such a relationship is a powerful resource in coping with the inescapable practice, management, and ethical problems."

Peer Support/Supervision Groups

Other psychotherapists prefer to formalize nurturance from colleagues by organizing peer supervision/support groups that regularly meet to discuss professional issues of concern. The best estimates are that 10–25% of practitioners attend a peer support, supervision, or consultation group on a regular basis (e.g., Lewis et al., 1988; Sherman & Thelen, 1998). In the words of one of our workshop participants: "I do a lot of self-care, but the best way to handle stressful situations created by encounters with difficult therapy clients is consultation with peers. That extra perspective and support usually means a lot."

Peer groups among clinicians have multiple advantages over mentor–protégé relationships (Gram, 1992). For one thing, they are often more readily available than seasoned mentors. For another, they are likely to be less expensive, if payment is expected of supervision. For still another, peer groups are advantageous in their implicit mutuality and nonhierarchical structure.

And peer groups typically serve multiple functions. These include providing a sense of community with other professionals, addressing unmet needs for appreciation, learning about practice management, sharing difficult cases and feelings, and receiving the support of fellow travelers. The content depends upon the goals of the group and the composition of the members but converges on providing mutual support in dealing with problematic cases, sources of stress, personal conflicts, and ethical matters. Research indicates that top expectations for peer consultation groups are to consider problem cases, discuss ethical and professional issues, and share information (Lewis et al., 1988).

All agree that peer groups must be carefully selected and structured to ensure trust and confidence. Confidentiality is the sine qua non for a successful group. "What is essential is that the group offer a safe, trusting arena for sharing of the stresses of personal and professional life" (Yalom, 2002, p. 254).

With or without a leader, peer groups are relatively easy to begin and nurture. You need a few dedicated members, a confidential setting, and a regular meeting time. Most groups contain 4 to 10 members and meet every 2 weeks to once a month for 2 hours per meeting. In rural or isolated areas, peer support is available via telephone or videoconferencing.

A specific form of peer supervision is the Balint group, named after the British psychoanalyst Michael Balint (1957). Here, a small group of clinicians create a safe and structured opportunity to explore what it is about a particular patient that touches the psychotherapist in certain ways. In an hour every other week, psychotherapists take turns presenting a patient and the dilemmas that treating them invoke. Then, colleagues take turns asking clarifying questions—not questioning your diagnostic or treatment decisions, but about how the psychotherapist experiences this particular patient. Thereafter the group offers, ideally in a nonjudgmental manner, a wide range of possible thoughts, conjectures, and feelings about what may be transpiring between the psychotherapist and the particular patient (Sternlieb, 2005).

The Balint group is a form of peer consultation, but differs from it as well. There is an identifiable group leader who facilitates the process and ensures that individual members are not challenged or criticized for their treatment decisions. The group's purpose is not to find solutions, offer advice, or present formal cases, as many peer consultation groups do. Instead, the Balint group strives to increase understanding of the patient's disorder and to offer divergent views on the therapist's response to the patient. In this respect, Balint groups are a hybrid of group therapy and peer consultation.

There are advantages and disadvantages to having peer groups meet at one's workplace. On the plus side, during work hours group members are all aware of the oppressive situation and demands of the setting, are familiar with each other, can provide on-site support, and can congeal the staff. On the downside, group meetings at the workplace can deteriorate into gripe sessions, can threaten confidentiality, might intensify existing rivalries, and can feel a little too close to home. We have been involved in and led both types of peer groups, some in-house and some from mixed-practice settings; we can recommend both.

The family therapy pioneer Carl Whitaker started "cuddle groups" for psychotherapists out of the recognition that peer support was invaluable. Therapists come together and support one another in their personal and professional growth. In fact, toward the end of his life, Whitaker participated for years in a cuddle group, exercising care to be just a member and facilitator, not the leader.

One of the participants in our self-care workshop summarized the results of her workshop experience like this: "I was inspired to get more strokes from work relationships. I talk to colleagues more during lunch instead of doing paperwork. I have also talked to my colleagues and supervisor about cuddle meetings to decompress. They received the idea warmly."

Peer groups are powerful vehicles; avail yourself of the opportunity or create your own group, if possible. Peer groups for practitioners serve as a personalized source of information and a forum for resolving specific ethical, legal, financial, and professional issues (Greenburg et al., 1985). To the extent that the psychotherapist can set aside concerns regarding professional reputation and competition, colleagues are an excellent source of encouragement and nurturance. One of our master clinicians described his group in this way:

"Our leaderless group of psychologists provides a format where each of us can express feelings and deal with life and work without trying to solve any specific problem or task, and without competing. It provides a point of balance for much of the rest of my life. We've been meeting for 90 minutes a week for several years. We deal with all kinds of stuff from the world of practice as well as personal things. All the way from which software to use for your practice to whether or not to take on a psychological assistant, the problems we face with bringing in a new psychologist into your practice, trying to build a career, what happens when people go out on their own and attempt to take clients with them whom you perceived as a part of your practice."

Clinical Teams

Can you imagine any health care treatment for a serious illness conducted by a single isolated practitioner? Neither can we. Serious disorders and intractable problems require multiple professionals working in coordination. Psychoses, borderline personality disorder, and similar impairing disorders call for a team approach.

Working as a clinical team can not only improve the patient's outcome but also nurture the psychotherapist. Team members may provide different services, be it individual therapy, group therapy, occupational therapy, pharmacotherapy, or residence supervision, thus sharing the burden. Teams can provide support, avoid insularity, and generate a sense of we-ness. One of our colleagues, Marsha Linehan (1993), specializing in the treatment of borderline and parasuicidal patients, likes to say that psychotherapists are not practicing her approach if they are not doing so as a team.

In this regard, we are ardent proponents of conducting cotherapy on occasion. It helps us remain fresh, avoid isolation, maintain contact with another therapist, and keeps us creative and challenged.

We are reminded here of an old Hasidic tale of the rabbi in a conversation with the Lord about heaven and hell (Yalom, 1975). "I will show you hell," said the Lord and led the rabbi into a room in the middle of which was a very big round table. The people sitting at it were famished and desperate. In the middle of the table there was a large pot of stew, enough and more for everyone. The smell of the stew was delicious and made the rabbi's mouth water. The people around the table were holding spoons with very long handles. Each one found that it was just possible to reach the pot to take a spoonful of the stew, but because the handle of the spoon was longer than a man's arm, each person could not get the food back into his or her mouth. The rabbi saw that their suffering was terrible.

"Now I will show you heaven," said the Lord, and they went into another room, exactly the same as the first. There was the same big round table and the same pot of stew. The people, as before, were equipped with the same long-handled spoons—but here they were well nourished and plump, laughing, and talking. At first the rabbi could not understand. "It is simple, but it requires a certain skill," said the Lord. "You see, they have learned to feed one another."

Whether in a dyad or in a larger team, let us learn to feed and nurture one another.

Staff

The physical and emotional isolation from colleagues, particularly in private practice, may be partially offset by nurturance from staff. Depending on the work site, psychotherapists may interact frequently with other staff—a receptionist, secretary, intake worker, or bookkeeper. They can provide an important source of contact and encouragement. They are often willing to partake in a few moments of casual conversation and shared humor that refresh the psychotherapist between appointments. Even those of us who work alone in the consulting office report that regular encounters with maintenance people, parking attendants, and other building tenants give us a chance to visit and build casual friendships that balance the intensity of a day filled with multiple therapy sessions. Don't overlook nonclinical people who physically surround you. They remind us that interpersonal interactions are more often about the price of tires than about existential angst!

Professionals in Community

Professionals located outside of the office are also vital sources of guidance and encouragement to psychotherapists. Physicians, lawyers, accountants, and the like not only provide professional advice but also are often willing companions for lunch and available partners for quick phone visits between sessions. Rely on them for business consultation, tax planning, legal advice, marketing, and so on. Those in allied helping professions offer mutual support in part because of the shared understanding that exists for what it takes to work with people—a mutual respect and care felt for other helping professionals, a kind of shared membership that creates natural ties. We suggest that you build relationships with professionals in the community who will assist and support you through a day of appointments. You'll find that they can be a meaningful source of nurturance.

Supervisors

What do psychotherapists rate as the most positive influences on their career development? Experience with patients, getting formal supervision or consultation, and getting personal therapy. Together, these three constitute what has been described as the major triad of positive influences on career development and on current development (Orlinsky & Rønnestad, 2005). Therapists accord more value to these interpersonal influences than to academic resources, such as taking courses, reading books or journals, or doing research.

Psychotherapists who regularly participate in formal supervision typically find it to be very helpful. One of our esteemed colleagues noted:

"Anything that I have a question about I know I can discuss at my next supervision appointment. It's helpful to have the chance to discuss issues with another therapist and get another opinion from someone with more experience that might see things differently. It's nice knowing that I always have some sort of safeguard. It increases my confidence a lot."

Supervision provides essential and realistic feedback. It is probably more important for those in solo practices, but also useful for those practicing in agencies and institutions.

It may sound obvious, but we argue not simply for supervision, but for *effective* supervision (Grosch & Olsen, 1994). Marginal supervision may be worse than none at all, and much agency-based supervision of seasoned practitioners is fairly unsatisfying, in our experience. Supervisors are assigned (not chosen), are selected on the basis of administrative talents (not necessarily clinical acumen), and may have a dual relationship (supervisor as well as evaluator). "How many people are going to reveal how stuck they feel with certain clients, or acknowledge that they are attracted to a client, to a supervisor who is then going to write their evaluation and has the power to fire them?" (Grosch & Olsen, 1994, p. 125). Simply put, the odds of getting quality clinical supervision at work may be slim.

If effective supervision is not available in house, then we heartily recommend that you (1) seek it privately and usually for a fee. Seek it from a seasoned and talented psychotherapist with no connection to your agency and with a compatible theoretical orientation and personal style. (2) Contract with a supervision group led by an experienced psychotherapist. (3) Join or create a peer supervision group. Or (4) do some combination of the preceding options.

In all instances, clinical supervision should address not only invariable case problems but also you as a person. What are the recurrent themes in difficult cases for you? Who do these patients remind you of? How do stressful clients leave you feeling? Good supervision is a safe haven for review of all that transpires in psychotherapy: problem cases, ethical quandaries, transference, countertransference, practice management, and reactivated conflicts from your personal history. Get what you need.

Mentors

There remains at least one more individual who can supply a nurturing relationship: the professional mentor. In that the practice of psychotherapy is a skill acquired through experiential learning, trainees quickly accept the need for mentoring during their training years (Betcher & Zinberg,

1988). Most realize that they will learn by "doing" under the oversight of a skilled, senior clinician who teaches the nuances of the psychotherapeutic encounter that cannot be learned from reading. What is not as widely recognized is the ongoing benefit of maintaining a mentoring relationship during later years of practice (Guy, 1987).

Virtually all surveys and interviews of successful psychotherapists wind up discussing the profound influence of professional elders or mentors (Rønnestad & Skovholt, 2001). The descriptions are powerful, passionate, and appreciative. The internalized influence continues in a contemporary and active way. We strongly recommend that each practitioners cultivate a strong attachment and positive investment with a professional mentor.

A mentor can offer guidance that is tailored to your individual personality and clinical needs, providing confrontation, nurturance, and direction in a manner that is more personal and informed than might be provided by a colleague. Contacts with the mentor can be conducted in person or by telephone as regularly scheduled events, or they can occur on a less frequent "as-needed" basis that is more like a consultation than a supervision appointment. In some cases, the mentor need only serve as a "touchstone" who is contacted primarily at times of critical career decisions or professional crisis. A trusted mentor serves an invaluable role throughout the professional life of the psychotherapist. It is regrettable that relatively few of us invest the time and energy necessary to maintain these mentoring relationships.

Clients

And now to a controversial source of nurturance for psychotherapists: clients. Few experienced practitioners are willing to openly divulge what most have actually experienced: clients can be powerful sources of support and encouragement in their lives.

Before we can comfortably consider this matter, let's first acknowledge the obvious concerns. Everyone agrees that the purpose of psychotherapy is to facilitate the client's relief and growth. The treatment contract specifies that the needs of the client take precedence over the needs of the therapist, at least to a reasonable extent. Professional ethics, legal precedence, and civil codes dictate the limits within which psychotherapists must operate. The therapy relationship exists to assist and support the client while enabling the psychotherapist to function in an effective, ethical manner.

At the same time, clients do provide therapists with special moments of nurturance and appreciation within a relationship that remains focused on the client's needs. It is simply not an either–or situation. It is essential, however, to be certain that this occurrence is not initiated, consciously or unconsciously, by therapist need. Simply put, clients are not there to meet the emotional needs of the psychotherapist. But respecting this fundamental principle does not prevent some clients from providing deep satisfaction to the psychotherapist.

A few examples will illustrate our point. Recall the discussion of intercurrent life events that bring the person of the psychotherapist into closer contact with the person of the client, as presented in Chapters 2 and 3. Research findings suggest that some clients discover and react to personal events in the life of the psychotherapist, such as marriage, pregnancy, divorce, loss of a loved one, illness or disability, and emotional distress (Guy, 1987; Guy et al., 1986; Guy, Poelstra, & Stark, 1989; Guy & Souder, 1986a, 1986b; Wahl et al., 1993). On some occasions, of course, patients react in hurtful, confused, or ambivalent ways. On other occasions, they respond with touching concern, care, and support. An appreciation of transference and the need to refocus on treatment goals may require that such expressions be thoughtfully scrutinized and interpreted. Nonetheless, there are real-life aspects to the treatment encounter, and client expressions of caring occasionally touch the soul of the psychotherapist in tender ways.

Two comments by master clinicians illustrate the thesis.

"I was really surprised by the concern and love expressed by some of my clients during my first pregnancy. Some of the women wanted to mother me, and some of the men became quite protective. We explored these feelings, and of course many were related to their own histories. Yet, I still appreciated their care; some of it seemed genuine, and that felt good to me."

Another told us of the "deep appreciation" for the cards and comments from patients when the local newspaper published an obituary of his father's death. "We only spent a few minutes of the session on their condolences—it is their therapy, not mine, after all—but their care was real and obvious. Moreover, it opened fruitful discussions about losses in their lives and about their feelings toward me. It was a pivotal moment for them and me."

Let us accept and be grateful for those moments when a client makes a comment, gives a compliment, smiles with gratitude, expresses concern, or even gives a touching (and appropriate) gift. In addition to its transferential elements, psychotherapy is at root a human relationship. It is permissible to acknowledge that the satisfactions resulting from conducting psychotherapy include the nurturance that comes from certain clients.

It's difficult to advise psychotherapists how to increase the nurturance that they receive from clients, since it is necessarily an occasional by-product of the practice of psychotherapy rather than a deliberate goal.

The need for nurturing relationships must be met in other ways, some yet to be described in this chapter. Nonetheless, we advise psychotherapists to accept the reality of this occurrence so that, despite the need to explore, interpret, reframe, or deflect many of the solicitous behaviors of clients, it is permissible to accept those few moments of genuine care and support expressed for the therapist. To graciously receive and gratefully acknowledge these moments reinforces a healthy reality for both therapist and client. These precious moments stand on their own merit and deeply touch the spirit of the psychotherapist.

Some psychotherapists confide that they structure their schedule with an eye toward alternating replenishing sessions with those that are more draining. To put it more bluntly, they intersperse their favorite or more satisfying clients among those who are more demanding, challenging, or deflating. This scheduling balance helps to avoid emotional exhaustion and overload. Patients should not be retained in treatment merely to support the practitioner; however, common sense forces us to recognize that some clients will be more enjoyable to work with than others. The psychotherapist intent on being effective and satisfied in her work will create a caseload mix that helps her remain focused, energetic, and optimistic throughout most of the day.

NURTURING RELATIONSHIPS OUTSIDE THE OFFICE

Now, we're on more comfortable ground. Most of us expect that our primary supply of nurturance will come from close relationships with people unrelated to the practice of psychotherapy. Spouses/partners, family, and friends provide our love and support. Love—both receiving it and giving it—heals. In Winnicott's sense, the therapist strives to create a holding environment for herself outside of the office where she can be soothed and nurtured (Kaslow & Farber, 1995).

Spouse/Partner

Regardless of one's marital status or sexual orientation, each individual feels a deep need to be known and loved by others. For many, this longing becomes focused on a particular individual or series of individuals, leading to lasting commitment and long-term relationships. Psychotherapists are no different. They marry at about the same rate as the general population (Wahl et al., 1993). Freud said long ago that the right marriage was an excellent alternative to a successful psychoanalysis.

The single highest rated career-sustaining behavior among psychotherapists is spending time with one's partner and family. It receives a mean rating of 6.15 on a 7-point scale (Stevanovic & Rupert, 2004). The second highest rated career-sustaining behavior is maintaining a balance between professional and personal lives. The highest rated self-care method among interns? Yep, you guessed it: close friends, significant others, and family as sources of support. It receives a mean rating of 4.3 on a 5-point scale (Turner et al., 2005).

In the best of situations, many emotional needs are met within the context of committed, loving relationships. A partner is able to provide near unconditional love and acceptance, deep understanding, and genuine encounter. When occupational hazards related to emotional constraint, isolation, and psychological mindedness are overcome, the clinician is finally free to participate with complete freedom in an intimate relationship of paramount importance. A spouse is able to keep the clinician in touch with inner needs, feelings, and longings that are set aside during a day of therapy sessions. Partners affirm our worth and dignity.

A mate is often best able to counter the assorted struggles of psychotherapy practice. On the one hand, for example, a mate can confront the grandiosity and sense of omnipotence that can grow over years of clinical work. This helps to prevent the therapist from accepting the distorted idealizations of clients as actual reality. On the other hand, a mate can provide a firm foundation of support and acceptance of the worries and struggles of clinical work. This helps the therapist to express hidden fears and hopes related to the "impossible profession." A nurturing partner has a significant impact on the professional confidence and competence of a psychotherapist.

Confidentiality must be considered here for a moment. We must remember that clients have the right to expect that their confidentiality will be protected by the psychotherapist (Pope et al., 1987). This includes preventing any inadvertent domestic slips of confidentiality, such as disclosing information to a spouse, unsecured documents at home, shared fax machine, or accidental revelation at the dinner table. Research suggests that, despite these ethical strictures, some psychotherapists do discuss job-related concerns with their partners (Tamura et al., 1994). Regrettably, this occasionally includes identifying details that violate client trust and risk accidental exposure of clinical material. Thus, limit discussion with a partner to feelings and thoughts that emerge in your inner world as a result of a psychotherapy session. This need not include any information about a client, nor need it involve a violation of professional ethics. Instead, the therapist shares her own internal process only as it relates to personal history and concerns.

Before leaving this topic, we would observe that psychotherapists tend to marry other psychotherapists at a surprising rate. In one national survey, about 20% reported that they married another psychotherapist (Guy, Tamura, & Poelstra, 1989). This pattern was even stronger among those married a second or third time. One is left to wonder whether such relationships increase the amount of understanding and nurturance that is shared between spouses, due to a commonality of experience. Several therapist couples (e.g., Weiss & Weiss, 1992) enthusiastically report that this has been the case for them during their careers. On the other hand, could it be that it is more difficult to reorient and re-enter the "real world" when both spouses spend considerable time in the world of multiple clients? Like all of life's adventures, a marital relationship between two psychotherapists must certainly be a mixed bag of assets and liabilities (Guy, Souder, Baker, & Guy, 1987). The first author of this book (JCN) has been happily married to another psychotherapist for more than 25 years, and the second author has remarried to a psychotherapist. So it can certainly be done!

Family Members

As in the case of a spouse/partner, there is something basic, something fundamental, about being known in a genuine fashion, unfettered by clinical distortions, by family members. Most psychotherapists appreciate their honest relationships with children, siblings, parents, and extended family. Within this world she is known as someone other than a psychotherapist. It's refreshing to get together with family who insist that the psychotherapist stop sounding so "therapeutic." They force us to come out from behind our clinical mask, prioritize life goals, and be genuine as humans.

A workshop participant tells us: "I spend time with my grandson every week now. . . . It allows me to get in touch with what is really important. The ladybug that rests on the window in my bathroom, which keeps us from taking our evening bath on time—or are we on time? Life seems just a little bit better now."

One of our master clinicians tells us:

> "My favorite way to decompress after psychotherapy is to play and exercise with my dog. In addition to providing a great workout and release of energy for both of us, spending time with a cherished dog can be an emotionally uplifting experience. The warmth and consistency of our relationship provides a wonderful antidote to the shifting emotions elicited during psychotherapy. My dog is always on time, willing to work, and gets along well with his family of origin."

Such self-care usefully reminds us that not all family members are human, nor even members of our biological family.

Children and pets have impressive ways of deflating the self-importance that results from spending many hours with clients who value our advice and opinions (Japenga, 1989). It is humbling indeed to be ignored, teased, disobeyed, and challenged by children who are all too familiar with our personal weaknesses. Yet, few have the ability to provide more meaningful moments of tender love and satisfaction than one's own children.

The research demonstrates that female therapists, compared to male therapists, tend to spend more time with families and friends (e.g., Coster & Schwebel, 1997; Kramen-Kahn & Hansen, 1998; Stevanovic & Rupert, 2004). Many factors probably account for this robust group difference, but we are concerned about men's tendencies to be less expressive or relational.

Many practitioners try to abide by the Family First Rule, namely, "All others get in line." But most of us slip, if not fall, in implementing the rule. And, in the interests of full disclosure, we two authors usually slip as well. One of us was fond of saying for years that there was an "unspoken" family rule of not traveling away from home more than once a month. The spouse, on more than one occasion, quipped that the rule was "unspoken *and* unkept!"

Even when home and not traveling, it is often difficult for psychotherapists to be good listeners after lengthy days of listening to patients. We are tempted to seek mostly admiration and appreciation from the family, as opposed to a healthy mix of admiration, criticism, and teasing. In the short run, we want others to listen to *us*; in the long run, we want the honesty of loving concern. If not, we begin to leave too much at the office and not bring enough of ourselves home.

Siblings, parents, and extended family can dole out steady supplies of nurturance throughout a lifetime. These are people who have known us perhaps since birth, including many years prior to our entry into the profession. This world of relationships is ideally a safe harbor of refuge in the midst of a busy career. Relatives are usually not invested in our particular clinical successes. In spite of the tendency of some to seek our advice on personal concerns or family conflicts, most family members continue a pattern of relating that predates the commencement of our psychotherapy career. This allows us to drop the role and accept the support of family members as genuine and without ulterior motives. There is purity to this nurturance that we intuitively understand. Within the limits imposed by family pathology, few people can make us feel as confident or secure. Yes, we hear you . . . and few people can make us feel as crazy!

Friends

Friends are good medicine. They share our deepest fears and most embarrassing foibles, hopefully with loving regard for both. Friends enjoy feelings of connection and acceptance, feelings not contaminated by the complications of marriage and family ghosts. One master clinician expressed it this way: "I find that my friends help me to lighten up. They make me set aside my role and be myself. They accept me for who I am, not for what I can do for them. My closest friends will always be there to help."

We bid you to keep your old civilian friends. Nonclinical friends offer a wider and healthier perspective on life. Fellow therapists can make fine friends, but having too many of them leads to equating life with "the job." Leave most of it—and them—at the office.

We all need friends, of course; yet, psychotherapists tend to have fewer and fewer friends over the course of their career (Cogan, 1977). This has led to speculation that perhaps, for better or worse, some affiliation needs are met through the practice of psychotherapy (Guy, 1987). Friendships outside the office also tend to be more difficult for male therapists raised to respect the male stereotype of the strong, solitary oak tree. "Real men don't need anybody" goes the common refrain. If you are tempted to rebut with the assertion that "male psychotherapists are different," please think again. Our culture rarely encourages intimate friendships among men.

As we discussed in Chapter 3, the reactions and expectations of casual friends sometimes make it difficult for the psychotherapist to escape the role of clinician. These individuals may not be a source of genuine encouragement, and interactions with them may be tainted by their expectations of psychotherapist rather than the actual person. It is the closer friend, committed to our well-being, who encounters the true person of the psychotherapist as a friend and companion.

These meaningful friendships are central sources of our strength. They remind us that most of life takes place outside of the consultation office. They help put things in perspective. Most people are not suicidal. Most people do not abuse children. Most are not crippled by anxiety and depression. Friends serve as reference points for this "normal" world, the world of which we are members. When invited, friends give honest feedback about the changes they note in the life and demeanor of the psychotherapist. As time passes, it is harder to find people who will be as honest as a true friend. Good friendships are worth the effort.

Colleague Assistance Programs

Should things turn nasty for your practice or career, reach out to spouses, family, friends, and, in addition, to organized state programs for assistance. Colleague Assistance Programs (CAP) provide resources for distressed clinicians and promote well-being. In the past, CAPs were designed for professionals in serious trouble; in the present, CAPs offer support and facilitation of professionals, including proactive self-care.

Approximately half of state psychological associations, for example, offer CAPs (American Psychological Association, 2006). Self-referrals are welcomed. All in the field agree that it is in the best interests of the public and the practitioner that we intervene early and often, before problems escalate into unmanageable monsters. We can help one another outside of the office instead of relying solely on punitive licensure boards or ethics bodies.

CAP programs offer multiple benefits to practitioners. These include advocacy, case monitoring, educational workshops, intervention/rehabilitation, liaison, outreach to professionals and students, peer support programs, referrals, consultation, support/information hotlines, and training workshops (Barnett & Hillard, 2001). Please proactively consider CAP, should trouble come calling.

Personal Mentors

Psychotherapists are meaning makers. We try to understand the derivative meanings associated with experiences, encounters, and events. This is usually true in the psychotherapist's personal life as well. We seek to make sense and meaning out of our own lives.

Most healers learn from mentors more experienced and powerful than themselves. We want to achieve the highest level of interpersonal effectiveness possible; we seek the nurturing direction of those who are successful and satisfied in their lives.

Psychotherapists often feel deeply committed to their lifelong growth. One path is to find a "life mentor" to support and guide us over many decades of life. Although this mentoring may include professional development, as discussed earlier in this chapter, the primary focus here is upon the development of a person, who happens to be simultaneously a psychotherapist. The life mentor may be a clergyperson, personal psychotherapist, favorite teacher, special relative, neighbor, or older friend or colleague. The role is gradually defined over time and usually acknowledged by both parties. Contact may be infrequent, but it is always meaningful.

The nurturance provided by a life mentor serves a unique purpose in the life of the psychotherapist. It is reassuring, curative, and motivating. It comes from a special person who is genuinely committed to the well-being of the psychotherapist, often without motive or guile. It is a gift that is thoughtfully given, and the spiritual aspects of the mentoring give a richness and depth of meaning that anchors the psychotherapist.

One of us (JDG) treasures a mentoring relationship with a favorite graduate professor that spans 30 years. This caring person has generously supported me through every major (and many minor) life challenges and career changes. It is invaluable self-care.

Personal Psychotherapist

Few have as strategic or vital an impact on the psychotherapist as her personal therapist. This individual alone has access to our most secret needs, fantasies, and experiences. The nurturance and insight gained from a personal psychotherapist is often without equal. In Chapter 10 we discuss this relational self-care in detail.

But let us here briefly present one compelling reason for seeking personal therapy or professional consultation away from the office when confronting a potentially litigious situation at the office. Whatever is said about such a legal matter might be used against the psychotherapist in subsequent legal proceedings (Ellis & Dickey, 1998). An expert on risk management in patient suicide (Bongar, 1991, p. 192) writes of the stark restraint of peer consultation in these situations:

> We must caution the reader: Any discussion with a colleague, or even with one's own family or friends, of the deceased patient's care is usually considered nonprivileged information that is open to the legal discovery process. That is, the plaintiff attorneys will subpoena colleagues and ask what was told to them about your concerns regarding the patient's suicide.

Thus, discussions of your feelings about potential misdiagnosis, treatment errors, or case mismanagement are best confined to the legally privileged contexts of legal consultation or personal psychotherapy. Be careful not to discuss your feelings about role or responsibility for any malpractice case or likely litigious case with colleagues or peers unless you are comfortable with those discussions becoming prosecution fodder in the courtroom.

IN CLOSING

Psychotherapists are people too. We are relational beings who find close, loving connections the most effective source of support, trust, and distress relief. The person of the therapist requires emotional nurturing, inside and outside the office, to avoid being a toxic sponge filled with clients' suffering. When confronted with occupational stress, our research-grounded recommendation is to tend and befriend, not fight or flight (Taylor et al., 2000).

Notice it is the *use* of nurturing relationships. Not simply having relationships available to you but actually *using* them for self-care. We have encountered the litany of psychotherapists' rationalizations for not using relationships—"I don't need to be pampered or nurtured," "I've worked though my oral dependency needs," or "No one truly understands my grind as a psychotherapist"—but find them unconvincing and transparent defenses. Of course, we need loving relationships. Psychotherapists are people too. The question is whether you give yourself the permission to be cared for, loved, and nurtured.

In her moving memoir *An Unquiet Mind*, psychologist Kay Redfield Jamison (1997) writes convincingly of the power of nurturing relationships in the treatment of her bipolar disorder: "For someone with my cast of mind and mood, medication is an integral element of this wall; without it, I would be constantly beholden to the crushing movements of a metal sea; I would, unquestionably, be dead or insane" (p. 215). And yet something more powerful was also operating in her life. She continues: "But love is, to me, the ultimately more extraordinary part of the breakwater wall: it helps to shut out the terror and awfulness, while, at the same time, allowing in life and beauty and vitality."

Following one of our self-care workshops, an experienced psychiatrist wrote of its effects on her: "I realized that all my self-care was solitary. I am a rather reclusive person anyway. The demands of psychotherapy combined with my personality have made for all solo activities—getting away from it all, so to speak. That is changing now." She allows herself to receive (as well as give) at home: "I'm off with my spouse and friends to dance and listen to music."

In our early years of presenting on psychotherapist self-care, we were disappointed with the specificity of what we were recommending. We felt that we were not concrete or specific enough in our recommendations. And perhaps you occasionally experience that feeling as you have been reading this chapter. But, over time, we have become convinced that presenting anything more specific is not only bad science (since the research does not indicate that any single method is more effective than another) but also disrespectful and presumptuous in addressing mental health professionals, who are themselves experts in behavior change. Yes, we know that the research on psychotherapist self-care indicates that the routine and sufficient use of nourishing relationships correlates with self-care effectiveness. But neither the research nor we can honestly tell you which path to nourishing relationships is available or preferable to you. Just be certain you are securing nurturing relationships in your life, somewhere, somehow.

So, follow the research evidence, the same evidence you probably faithfully recite to your patients. Research documents that your age, gender, income, job title, and even your health have small effects on your life satisfaction or happiness (Myers, 1993, 2000). The largest determinant of happiness appears to be a supportive network of close relationships. Luxuriate in your relationships, feel the connection, pursue the reciprocity of nurturance.

We need an array of relationships outside of the consulting office to ensure a balanced, satisfying life. Not only is a full complement of trusted friends and family desirable for a fulfilling existence, but psychotherapists rely on these relationships when assessing their clinical competency. Our research shows that clinicians expect family and friends to identify professional impairment or incompetence related to emotional distress or advancing age well before patients or colleagues become aware of their existence (Guy, Poelstra, & Stark, 1989; Guy, Stark, et al., 1987). Clinicians expect these individuals to confront them, and they report that they rely on their judgment and feedback when deciding to reduce or terminate clinical practice. Families and friends are the therapist's primary sources of nurturance and support; their impact on both personal life and professional practice is beyond measure.

We recommend that you give careful thought to the sources of nurturance in your life. Are they adequate? Is there variety and balance? How can they be utilized more effectively? These are among the most critical self-assessments that you can conduct when evaluating how to become more effective at "leaving it at the office."

Coming full circle, we conclude with a reminder from Flannery O'Connor's short story "The Lame Shall Enter First" that began this chapter. We implore you to become a good Sheppard, not a sacrificial lamb. Become the bounty-ful and boundary-ful clinician devoted simultaneously to self *and* to service.

SELF-CARE CHECKLIST

✓ Self-assess your peer support at the office. How does it fare? In one study of well-functioning psychologists (Coster & Schwebel, 1997), peer support emerged as the highest priority.

✓ Identify the three most nurturing people in your life. What can you do to increase the amount of support you receive from them?

✓ Insist on sufficient alone time. Do you know what to do with it when it's available?

✓ Pursue ongoing nurturance at the office with your clinical colleagues; take lunch, conversations, and walks with one another.

✓ Join or organize a peer support, supervision, or cuddle group.

✓ Participate in clinical teams and periodically conduct cotherapy to keep yourself fresh and vital.

✓ Seek nurturance from professionals in the community for both business assistance and collegial friendships.

✓ Develop arrangements for ongoing supervision or consultation. If it is unavailable or ineffective at your employment setting, then purchase it.

✓ Determine which clients "recharge your batteries" and brighten your day. Within the constraints of ethics and transference, structure your daily schedule and review your caseload to ensure that you see some of these patients on a daily basis.

✓ Identify the interpersonal gratifications you receive from favorite clients and what happens following termination with them.

✓ Name your most significant mentor during your career. How are your needs for mentoring being met today?

✓ Follow the evidence: the highest-rated career-sustaining behavior for psychotherapists is spending time with one's spouse/partner and friends.

✓ Try to include phone calls, lunches, and breaks in your workday several times each week to provide contact with family and friends.

✓ Maintain your old, civilian friends who keep you grounded in life outside of clinical work.

✓ Utilize your family-of-origin relationships to help you reality test and to confront your grandiosity.

✓ Beware if your friendships are becoming fewer in number or diminishing in significance over the years of professional practice. Take corrective action if necessary.

✓ Take advantage of Colleague Assistance Plans, should practice troubles come your way.

✓ Something may be amiss if you are habitually giving out far more nurturance than you are receiving. Seek a personal mentor or personal therapist to remedy the imbalance.

✓ When confronted with occupational stress, tend and befriend, rather than fight or flight.

RECOMMENDED READING

American Psychological Association. (2006). *Advancing colleague assistance in professional psychology.* Washington, DC: Author. Available at *www.apa.org/practice/acca_monograph.pdf.*

Balint Groups. (2006). Available online at *familymed.musc.edu/balint/index.*

Guy, J. D. (2000). Holding the holding environment together: Self-psychology and psychotherapist care. *Professional Psychology: Research and Practice, 31*, 351–352.

Norcross, J. C. (Ed.). (2002). *Psychotherapy relationships that work.* New York: Oxford University Press.

Scott, C. D., & Hawk, J. (1986). *Heal thyself: The health of health care professionals.* New York: Brunner/Mazel.

Yalom, I. D. (2002). *The gift of therapy.* New York: HarperCollins.

CHAPTER 6

Setting Boundaries

"How can I cut my hours down to 40 and walk away feeling justified? This really nails the dilemma for most of us. How to hold the line, shorten sessions, just say no, etc. In a nutshell, I think it requires a profound cognitive-emotional shift—helpers have needs too. Can I say 'no,' 'enough,' 'good enough for now' and still feel professional, effective, and ethical?"

Thus wrote one of our workshop participants in reflecting on the fundamental conflict in her self-care. How do we balance the needs of patients with the needs of ourselves? How do we set consistent boundaries that humanely serve the interests of all involved?

The process of clarifying and balancing interpersonal relationships lies at the heart of the psychotherapeutic endeavor. Regardless of theoretical orientation, this process is one of the most complex and challenging of conducting psychotherapy. It can also become a primary source of distress among psychotherapists, particularly when confusion exists regarding roles and expectations. Psychotherapists who have difficulty establishing clear, reasonable boundaries will almost certainly have trouble leaving it at the office.

In a general sense, *boundary* implies a limit or territory that is not to be violated. In a psychological sense, boundary denotes maintenance of a distinction between the self and the other—what is within bounds and what is out of bounds. Some psychotherapists, especially those of psychoanalytic origin, prefer the term *therapeutic frame*. By whatever name, the primary function of boundaries is to provide a safe and predictable environment for the patient to work and for the therapist to render effective care.

We are in the mainstream in suggesting that therapists manage daily boundaries of psychotherapy for the benefit of their patients and for themselves. Being regular, predictable, and punctual does not replicate the chaotic life history that many patients bring to treatment. The holding environment and the comforting structure of office policies reassure patients. Boundaries serve to maintain safety and integrity in the psychotherapeutic process (Epstein, 1994).

At the same time, we are mindful that efforts to consistently manage boundaries can deteriorate into rigid, even punitive, behavior that causes ruptures and threatens the therapeutic alliance. While we advocate in this chapter for setting boundaries, we also advocate for reasonable flexibility. The results of survey research indicate that most patients make relatively few requests about extending boundaries and that psychotherapists accommodate the requests most of the time (Johnston & Farber, 1996). Such practice suggests a spirit of good will, flexibility, and collaboration. We try to allow flexibility within limits—the bend-but-don't-break rule. Accordingly, in the following pages, we hope that our insistence on setting and maintaining boundaries is interpreted as consistent and predictable, yet flexible.

Not surprisingly, research bears out the self-care value of clear yet flexible boundaries. Psychotherapists who maintain clear boundaries feel less stressed by patient's psychopathology and suicidal threats. By contrast, therapists with greater fusion tendencies experience more stress from patients' pathology and suicidality and report more professional doubt about maintaining the therapeutic relationship (Hellman, Morrison, & Abramowitz, 1987a). Again, we encounter the inescapable interaction of the therapist's personality and the hazards of the work.

Setting boundaries consistently emerges in the research as one of the most frequently used *and* one of the most highly effective self-care principles. In one study of boundary behaviors used to prevent distress and impairment (Sherman & Thelen, 1998), 72% of psychotherapists scheduled breaks during the day, 59% kept their caseload at a specific level, and 56% refused certain types of clients. These are impressive numbers, but in an ideal self-care future we hope these numbers would top 90%!

In this chapter, we consider the self-care imperative of setting boundaries both at the office and away from the office. On this point there is universal agreement. A common thread among both passionately committed (Dlugos & Friedlander, 2001) and master (Skovholt & Jennings, 2004) psychotherapists is their insistence on creating boundaries between their professional and nonprofessional lives. The master clinicians interviewed for this book are unanimous in declaring that boundaries must be established to ensure the well-being and relationships of the psychotherapist. In fact, establishing clear boundaries was the most frequently cited self-care strategy of our master clinicians.

SETTING BOUNDARIES AT THE OFFICE

Boundaries at the office encompass an intersecting network of role definitions: what is in bounds and what is out of bounds for the psychotherapist, the patient, their therapy relationship, colleagues, family, and friends. Let's consider each in turn with an eye toward psychotherapist self-care.

Defining the Role of the Psychotherapist

It is of paramount importance that the psychotherapist understand her role. She must recognize personal strengths and limitations and establish clearly defined boundaries (Gregory & Gilbert, 1992; Pope, 1991). This is done in a number of ways, but begins with and requires self-awareness.

For starters, how do you characterize your role in the treatment process? This is largely an expression of the practitioner's theoretical orientation and personal style. Some psychotherapists see themselves as educators, who seek to instruct clients in the complicated nature of human relationships and the process of behavior change. If so, this will partially determine your style within the context of the treatment relationship. The educative psychotherapist will most likely be quite active, freely self-disclosing and instructing the client by providing content and skills. Psychotherapists who see themselves as "prophets" in the lives of clients will exhort and encourage them to higher levels of functioning, convincing and confronting them when necessary. Supportive clinicians who view their role as that of comforter and facilitator will probably listen more, talk less, and seek to understand and nurture the inner worlds of the clients. Analytically inclined psychotherapists will engage in reconstructive work that requires a more reflective style of observation and interpretation.

The psychotherapist who understands her role, as defined by theoretical orientation and personal style, will have an easier time clearly communicating this persona and professional service to the client. This process will help shape expectations and reduce misunderstanding and disappointment. This may be as basic as deciding how many total hours the psychotherapist will work each week, which nights (if any) she will be available for appointments, and how many breaks will be necessary throughout the day to ensure quality care. It will also be important to decide how available the clinician will be for telephone contacts, crisis sessions, and

multiple appointments per week. All of these decisions require an awareness of the overall relationship between the psychotherapist's professional
practice and personal life.

The more the psychotherapist can establish necessary boundaries,
the easier it will be for her to commit to their maintenance. A master therapist put it this way:

> "I make it clear that I keep clinical work in my office during my work-
> day and try not to bring it home with me. My family time is family
> time, leisure time is leisure time, and work time is work time. I set
> those boundaries in my own mind to try to keep clinical work in the
> office. I have to make a decision to not worry about a client who is
> telling me he or she is doing something that is putting them at risk."

Consider the number of hours a practitioner is willing to work each
week. The goal of some therapists is to do as much psychotherapy as possible per week—that is, until they begin to "drift away" during sessions,
offer mechanical responses, or are unable to physically tolerate another
session. We suggest that the goal should be doing as much therapy as you
can do *well*. Everyone has a different limit; Albert Ellis, one of the fathers
of cognitive-behavioral therapy (CBT), famously does 60 hours a week,
while others max out at about 30 contact hours. The goal is not more psychotherapy but better psychotherapy. Determining your own workload
should be made by observing and honoring your feelings. If you find
yourself becoming irritable, distracted, and exhausted during many work-
days, then please honor those feelings and take corrective remedies.

Most of us are socialized to work to capacity (100%) or above capacity
(110%). We recommend working under capacity (90%) so that emergencies, family demands, and self-care can be accommodated and, indeed,
built into the weekly schedule.

Those of us who measure our "success" by the fullness of our
appointment book and the number of sessions scheduled per day can
come to regard unanticipated or unscheduled free time as a blemish to be
hidden as quickly as it appears (Penzer, 1984). How easy it is to skip lunch
in order to see another patient!

Overwork is a curse of our time and simultaneously a badge of honor
(Grosch & Olsen, 1994). Listen to a busy practitioner "complain" about
her full schedule and overwork: it is a mix of grumbling *and* bragging.
What an important, esteemed healer I am! Here is where the masked narcissism of many psychotherapists reveals itself.

This is a paradox of self-care, as we noted in Chapter 1: many of us
embark on helping careers out of a genuine concern for others but also a
need to be appreciated by them (Grosch & Olsen, 1994). We must realistically assess and continually monitor our need for appreciation, the deep

desire to be liked and admired. Such motives may easily drive us to over-work.

Consider, too, the nature of session fees. In the ratio of length of professional training to average income, mental health professionals occupy the bottom rungs. Conducting psychotherapy as a licensed professional requires at least a master's degree. How many MAs and MSWs outearn MBAs? Or PhDs outearning MDs? Psychologists, in particular, are at real risk of becoming the health care professionals with the longest training (average of 6 years postbaccalaureate) but the lowest incomes. We are in real danger of becoming a masochistic profession in which we take care of the legitimate needs of others but not of ourselves.

The psychotherapy literature has been hesitant to talk about money (Rappoport, 1983). The profession has come out of the dark more recently, given the ravages of managed care; but money remains a deeply ambivalent subject to most mental health professionals. We suffer from moral uneasiness about profiting from the emotional distress of others.

Still, boundaries demand livable wages and a reasonable return on the investment that is required to become a psychotherapist. Income deserves to be addressed for the major dimension and reality element it is. None of us enters the profession solely for the money, for most of our occupational rewards are nonmonetary (see Chapter 3). However, we deserve a "good enough" income.

And consider how some psychotherapists deal with patients late for their scheduled appointments. We frequently encounter therapists who will see patients for their entire scheduled time (30 or 50 minutes, for instance) even if the patient (or couple) has arrived late for the appointment. As a result, subsequent appointments are pushed back for the remainder of the day. These therapists seem to be always running late and perpetually exhausted (Boylin & Briggie, 1987). Our advice is to maintain the time boundaries; see patients for only their scheduled time and only extend appointments on rare occasions if warranted.

Consider as a final example of psychotherapists' role definition the matter of availability outside of sessions. Each therapist must decide what she can realistically offer, keeping in mind how committed one is to her personal needs versus those of the client. The following disclosure by one of our master clinicians demonstrates one way of handling this conflict:

"I encourage people to contact me only in true emergencies. Sometimes we talk specifically about when it is appropriate to call my beeper. When there are clinical issues that require their calling me, I label it clearly. I try to be prompt and clear about telephone calls that I get and return. I also try to be on time with sessions. I let [clients] know that I don't give extra time in sessions unless there seems to be an extraordinary reason."

Practitioners naturally differ in their policies for out-of-session contacts. On one end, some of our colleagues maintain only a telephone answering machine with a message advising their patients to go to the emergency room in a crisis. In the middle are those who maintain a beeper, cell phone, or answering service but are clear that they frequently cannot be reached. On the other end are those who take calls 24/7.

We offer no self-care advice on which of these policies is optimal for your particular circumstances, but would offer four self-care caveats. First, it is a decision that should be made by you, not your patients. Second, it is a decision that should be clearly communicated to patients and potential patients. Third, when possible, limit your out-of-session exposure to crises by minimizing on-call circumstances, referring patients to the emergency room, and dividing calls among fellow professionals in your agency or in your office. When on your own time, surrender the beepers and the cell phones at the door! And fourth, thoughtfully select patients and clinical circumstances that fit with your on-call availability. Practitioners who are not generally available and who do not have backup arrangements should not be taking on chronically suicidal patients in their practices, for one obvious example.

Exceptions are the rule in clinical practice, of course. Circumstances may occasionally demand that the clinician extend herself beyond stated limitations in order to assist a client undergoing extraordinary difficulties. Sliding-scale fees, pro bono sessions, extra sessions, late-day appointments, and telephone contacts may be necessary from time to time. However, in such situations the therapist should remain in the position of deciding the appropriateness of the exceptions and should clearly demarcate them as exceptions.

Combining your personal style, theoretical orientation, and individual resources into a clearly defined persona as a psychotherapist is a gradual process. It's important to repeatedly assess your needs and priorities in order to be clear with your clients as to what you offer—and do not offer—as part of the treatment contract. Establish a personal policy and a method to determine whether a particular boundary has been crossed. Boundary violations are frequently realized only after the fact; it is a recursive process of trial and error that requires vigilant self-monitoring on your part. By understanding, monitoring, and maintaining your boundaries, you will be better able to communicate them unambiguously and unapologetically to your clients.

Defining the Role of the Client

Few would disagree that there must be a clear set of expectations established for psychotherapy clients (Gutheil, 1989). Ethical principles governing the practice of psychotherapy require informed consent, which includes discussing the role of the client and securing agreement on terms mutually before commencing treatment.

For the psychotherapist, however, the fecal matter hits the boundary fan in trying to honor both patients' desires and self-preservation. The decision to give 15 extra minutes to a patient means you leave 15 minutes late from the office or arrive 15 minutes late for your child's piano recital. Research has no easy answers here, other than that achieving the right balance is an ongoing process requiring continuous self-monitoring, judicious compromises, and consistent boundaries.

Good practice demands that psychotherapists help clients verbalize their role expectations early in the treatment process and then reach an explicit consensus. Goal consensus and collaboration do contribute to effective psychotherapy (Tryon & Winograd, 2002).

At the same time, good self-care demands that psychotherapists communicate and maintain their boundaries. For example, one's fees for services always need to be defined. Is the fee to be paid in full at the time of the session? Should the fee be paid at the beginning or end of the session? Is it allowable for the client to carry a balance in his or her account? If so, is there a limit to how much the client can owe the therapist before treatment will be discontinued? How will insurance reimbursements be handled? All these arrangements should be specified in advance of commencing services.

Similarly, policies regarding the scheduling of sessions are discussed at the outset of treatment and maintained throughout unless mutually revised. Will the sessions be weekly? What will be their length? Will they include anyone besides the client, such as might occur in couples, family, or group psychotherapy? How will late arrivals be handled? The cancellation policy must be discussed so that the client knows the expectations of the psychotherapist regarding missed sessions, rescheduling, and breaks due to illness or vacations. The psychotherapist's policy regarding telephone contacts between sessions must be explained, including any associated costs to the client.

Increasingly, psychotherapists are gravitating toward the use of informed consent forms that contain many of these important policies. The forms may be handed to clients to read, discuss, and then sign as a written treatment contract or, alternatively, may be used by practitioners as a template for topics to be covered during the initial sessions (see Pomerantz & Handelsman, 2004, and Harris & Bennett, 2005, for sample forms). We have used both methods in our practices with success. In both methods, the form contains information regarding appointments, fees, cancellations, billings, payments, extrasession contacts, crisis contacts, release of information to third parties, managed care reimbursement, HIPAA regulations, exceptions to confidentiality, and so on. Preliminary research shows that informed consent forms yield many practical benefits to the patient—more information, more comfort, a more favorable impression of the therapist—and to the therapist—feeling more thorough in covering essential topics, feeling more protected in a legal and ethical sense (Sullivan, Martin, & Handelsman, 1993). Despite these findings and despite our positive experiences with them in our own practice, we are concerned that lengthy, legalistic forms may misconvey the essence of psychotherapy.

At the conclusion of the therapy relationship, expectations for the future must be discussed. In particular, what if any contact will be permitted between the client and the therapist? Who will initiate the contact? It should not be assumed that there is a mutual understanding and agreement on this issue until it has been discussed. One of our studies revealed a great deal of variation on posttermination contact (Guy et al., 1993). Although 86% of psychotherapists surveyed avoided social contact with former clients, 78% allowed the exchange of letters, 79% permitted telephone contact, and 93% encouraged future therapy sessions when needed. In nearly all of these cases the subsequent contact was initiated by the client. For the conscientious psychotherapist, there are ways in which treatment relationships never really end. A meaningful discussion of these issues at the time of termination will lessen the possibility of unrealistic expectations or patient disappointment.

Defining the Boundaries of the Treatment Relationship

Having clarified the respective roles of the psychotherapist and the client, it is essential to delineate the nature of the psychotherapy relationship early in the treatment process. This helps to focus psychotherapy in order to foster the alliance, to increase its effectiveness, and to reduce misunderstanding regarding the boundaries that are to be a part of this intimate encounter.

One prevalent assumption of clients, particularly clients new to the process, is that the psychotherapist is going to fix, heal, or "treat" them. Patients overly socialized in the medical model expect to be the relatively passive recipient of services unilaterally dispensed by an expert doctor who is largely in charge and responsible for the outcome of treatment.

Such a patient perspective unfortunately fits with a conventional view of therapist distress and burnout as caused by the grueling nature of the work and the experience of failure. The emotional exhaustion and intrapsychic depletion characteristic of burnout can result from over-responsible therapists who too readily assume responsibility for their clients' lives or feel they need to save or rescue them. Therapists quickly become drained, overburdened, and soon feel underappreciated by all. This often represents a boundary (and thinking) problem: over-responsibility.

An alternative view is that we become dispirited, not because we are failures, but because our hierarchical view of therapy emphasizes our ideas and actions while according little attention to our clients' perspectives. When we assume the one-up position of expert, then we become responsible for change.

Instead, we emphasize early in therapy our mutual responsibility for both the process and the outcome. Psychotherapy demands a highly collaborative process, beginning with our thinking and ending with behavior within session. We discuss shared responsibility for change. Yes, we are experts in some respects, but a "fellow traveler" in most respects.

One technique for facilitating shared responsibility is "transparency" (White, 1997), in which the therapist owns personal ideas and communicates possible frailties and empathic lapses to clients. We (the authors writing this book, for example) might acknowledge to the patient, that "our backgrounds as heterosexual white men may not allow us to fully appreciate your experiences as an African-American woman. We may convey feelings or share ideas that make more sense to a man than to a woman. Should that occur, please let us know" (McCollum, 1998). Active collaboration sets boundaries and reinforces mutual responsibilities for the change process and treatment outcomes.

An administrator made several boundary commitments following our self-care workshop. To wit: "I will stop 'fixing' everything. Let other people make mistakes, and don't engage in prevention or fixing if they do. Don't do everything I know how to do, even though it's not my job, just because others know I know how to do it. It's the only way for people and institutions to learn." Sharing responsibility with patients (and with colleagues) is a boundary fix.

Once the relationship is defined as a shared responsibility, the challenge is to protect that relationship. To do so requires a mutual commitment to its maintenance and integrity. Specifically, psychotherapy must not be compromised by blending it with other possible interactions. For example, the psychotherapist and client must not enter into other types of relationships together. They are not free to become business partners, professional colleagues, friends, or lovers (Pope, 1991, 1993; Pope, Sonne, & Holroyd, 1993; Stake & Oliver, 1991). It is not appropriate for them to meet in other contexts that require additional roles that may conflict with those of client and psychotherapist (Borys & Pope, 1989; Pope, Tabachnick, & Keith-Spiegel, 1988). To work, play, study, or live together would most likely undermine the nature of the psychotherapy relationship. There is wide recognition among mental health organizations that it is necessary to avoid multiple role conflicts that would prove detrimental to the patient. The clearer the boundary is in this regard, the more effective the treatment will be.

Our master clinicians were nearly unanimous in communicating often with clients about the boundaries to be respected. Numerous personal examples were given regarding the importance of keeping the professional roles separate from personal roles outside the office. The following is typical:

> "I had a patient who was celebrating a birthday. She wanted to invite me to the party, and she was hoping that I would go. We talked about it, and what it would mean to her if I did go. By helping her describe what it would mean, she got to issues that were important to her in the therapeutic process. It reminded her of things that she needed from her mother and father and did not get. By keeping myself in the room with the patient rather than going to a social event, it was a useful therapeutic re-doing. Had I gone to the party, it would have been a therapeutic disappointment. It helps me to set boundaries with patients, and it gives me more confidence in the treatment. I don't touch patients, talk much about myself, or talk to family members of patients. I don't socialize with patients. I have a whole constellation of boundaries that I set."

This advice converges with the research on extrasession contacts with our psychotherapy patients. For example, about 60% of psychotherapists never accept an invitation to a client's party or social event and about a third rarely do so (Pope et al., 1987). We fall squarely between the never and rarely camp. Frequent social excursions can contaminate the therapeutic relationship, violate a nonsexual boundary, and interfere with the sanctity of a therapist's private life. At the same time, we do make exceptions when the patient's health and circumstances seem to require it.

In a nutshell, maintaining boundaries entails saying "no" when deemed to be in the interest of the patient's treatment and/or in the interest of the psychotherapist's effectiveness. Herb Freudenberger (1983), father of the term *burnout*, has written eloquently of the need for health practitioners to say "no." Protect yourself from the high cost of success; strive not to be perfect or to cling to the ego ideal of perfect, compulsive care giver. It is not your job to meet everyone's needs. Your goal is always to get people to push their own wheelchairs, even if they are never able to walk again (Berkowitz, 1987).

Saying "no" will necessarily come in many guises. These include:

- "No" to patient requests for routine exceptions to your policies regarding no-shows, cancellations, and unpaid bills.
- "No" to patients trying to extend the length of sessions and making emergency calls that are not emergencies.
- "No" to potential patients who seek treatment for disorders or conditions (e.g., psychotic, personality-disordered) that you are unable or unwilling to provide.

- "No" to accepting at-risk or suicidal patients into your practice when you are already stretched thin.
- "No" to an agency's excessive, even inhumane, working conditions. It is in the nature of organizations to keep asking for better performance, but it is the practitioner's personal responsibility to decline inhumane demands (Lyall, 1989). The antidote is good, old-fashioned boundaries: assertively notifying management of the excessive burden, assertive discussions about reasonable pace, and the responsibility to educate others about workload expectations.
- "No" to referral sources who request that you perform activities, such as forensic work, child custody evaluations, or hospital consultations that you do not desire to perform.
- "No" to managed care organizations that undervalue your services and pay egregiously low rates and require extensive, unreimbursed paperwork.
- "No" to the institutionalization of mental health care that attempts inappropriate incursions into the psychotherapy you offer.

Let us be crystal-clear here: We are not advocating remaining entrenched in old therapy models or avoiding newer, briefer treatments. On the contrary, it behooves us all to keep updated on more effective and efficient means to alleviate human suffering. What we urge you to avoid is practicing in ways you do not believe in—ways that undermine your ethics and integrity—since they add inordinate stress and compromise patient care (Bromfield, 1996). For example, our ethics and integrity are assaulted by adopting a purely medical model, overemphasizing DSM diagnoses, losing track of the human relationship, and employing "any willing" licensed therapist.

Say "no" as a matter of integrity. The cost to your soul is simply too high.

Many psychotherapists experience difficulty in asserting themselves in professional settings, particularly with their clients. Table 6.1 presents eight professional rights that assertive therapists take to heart (Janzen & Myers, 1981). While we would phrase some of these rights differently, their principal value is in reminding us of our inherent right, our perfect right, to say "no" at times.

Phrased more positively, assertively maintaining boundaries means remaining true to yourself, your moorings, and your vocation (Norcross, 2005a). Relentlessly define who you are and what you do. Know and accept your limits.

Speaking of limits, we enthusiastically recommend that psychotherapists more frequently transfer difficult cases—either for a second opinion or evaluation or the entire treatment—to a colleague (Kaslow & Schulman, 1987). A transfer is indicated whenever the case becomes prolonged, inef-

TABLE 6.1. A Professional Bill of Rights for Psychotherapists

1. Psychotherapists have the right to say "no" to their clients.
2. Psychotherapists have the right not to become emotionally involved with their clients.
3. Psychotherapists have the right not to like their clients.
4. Psychotherapists have the right to actively avoid their patients' feelings (when appropriate).
5. Psychotherapists have the right to prevent clients from interfering in their personal lives.
6. Psychotherapists have the right to disagree with their clients.
7. Psychotherapists have the right to be less than technically perfect with their clients.
8. Psychotherapists have the right to have limits in their areas of professional expertise.

Note. Based on and adapted from Janzen and Myers (1981). Copyright 1981 by the American Psychological Association. Adapted by permission.

ficacious, a poor client–therapist match, a shaky therapeutic alliance, or simply outside of one's competence. Such a transfer can be interpreted as a sign of strength and wisdom, not failure. And all ethics codes prohibit us from practicing beyond our sphere of competence and remind us to consider transfer whenever services are not proving efficacious. In addition, transfer should be considered when the patient's struggles and circumstances are too similar to the therapist's life. The terminal illness of a close family member, a recent death or divorce, or the chronic illness of a child are prominent examples. Nonacceptance or transfer of patients at such times "represents a sensitive and humble awareness of one's limitations and the placing of the patient's needs for efficacious treatment above one's own for a busy therapy schedule" (Kaslow & Schulman, 1987, p. 92).

Maintaining proper boundaries means not only saying "no" but also saying "I don't know." It's honest, avoids defensiveness, and confronts your perfectionist tendencies head-on. We simply cannot know everything!

Defining Relationships with Colleagues and Staff

Just as it is essential to understand, communicate, and maintain the boundaries of the treatment relationship, it is also useful to clarify the relationships that exist among colleagues (Tabachnick, Keith-Spiegel, & Pope, 1991). The psychotherapist will experience a number of potential role relationships with her colleagues. In some cases, she may assume the role of peer, with all the mutual respect and support that this implies. In other relationships, she may behave more like a parent, rival sibling, or friend. Obviously, this process is not restricted to psychotherapists; it is true of all work relationships. However, the emotionally rich and psychologically potent world of the psychotherapist seems to exaggerate the problems normally encountered with colleagues in a work context.

This phenomenon becomes particularly acute when the roles are compromised by a blurring of boundaries (Slimp & Burian, 1994). For example, it is universally recognized as unethical for a clinical supervisor to become a lover of his or her supervisee (Tabachnick et al., 1991). The role of supervisor or colleague also generally precludes the formation of a personal psychotherapy relationship with supervisees. In some cases, the administrator of a clinic may find it difficult to assume the role of peer and friend as a result of the power differential associated with his or her "parenting" role.

Psychotherapist–staff relationships also become tricky and strained if boundaries are not maintained. Staff are part friends to psychotherapists, part of the clinical team, and yet frequently employees or direct reports to psychotherapists. The blurring of roles and the relationship elements frequently confuses staff members not formally trained in graduate coursework. We and others have found it useful to take an hour periodically to discuss openly the therapist–staff relationship.

Such relationships can be further strained when psychotherapists delegate nonclinical duties to staff, who frequently experience it as "getting more work dumped" on them. Psychotherapists are wise to delegate such tasks and to free up their time and energy to concentrate on what they uniquely do best. Indeed, we encourage you to delegate all nonclinical work such as filing, xeroxing, word processing, scheduling appointments, billing, and related office tasks. Even if you personally pay for it, delegate to others whatever runs counter to your skills and interests. See an extra patient per week and eliminate 3 hours of drudgery!

All told, we urge you to monitor and maintain your boundaries with colleagues. Defining the nature of these professional relationships, whether they are to be sources of nurturance or professional advice, will help you negotiate the complexities related to boundaries and expectations.

Defining Boundaries with Family and Friends

Family and friends are not usually direct participants in the professional world of the psychotherapist. They are not present during psychotherapy sessions, they do not meet clients, and they do not assist with the delivery of services. Confidentiality requires that the clinician not share the identities and disclosures of clients with them. This leaves family and friends outside of the clinical experience of the practitioner. One of our master psychotherapists described it this way: "My kids don't really know what I do for a living. It's hard to explain it to them, and I can't really show them. They've seen the office; they know I talk and listen to people who are unhappy or have problems. But they really can't understand why I get paid for this. After all, I do the same for them at home all the time . . . and not always very effectively!"

Without considerable effort, there is little opportunity for spontaneous phone calls, personal visits, and short breaks with friends and family during the typical workday. The clinician spends most of her time with clients, many of whom are in distress. Moreover, since the focus on the client is often intense and engrossing, there is little opportunity for the therapist to think about personal relationships during a long day at the office.

Find ways to bridge this gap. Deliberately schedule lunch appointments and visits with friends and family during the workday. When possible, telephone loved ones between appointments.

SETTING BOUNDARIES AWAY FROM THE OFFICE

In order to effectively disengage and leave it at the office, the psychotherapist must realize that clearly defined boundaries are also necessary outside of the office. One of our master clinicians commented in an interview:

> "I make it clear that I keep clinical work in my office during my workday and try not to bring it home with me. I avoid talking about what's happening in my clinical work with my family or with other people, feeling that family time is family time and leisure time is leisure time and work time is work time. I set those boundaries in my own mind to try and keep clinical work in the office."

Establishing secure boundaries is essential in maintaining some distance between a therapist's personal life and professional practice. Doing so will require a thoughtful attempt to define the roles of several significant people who populate the world of the psychotherapist, beginning with the therapist herself.

The Psychotherapist outside the Office

It is not enough to know "who you are" at the office; you must also know who you are when you've left and gone home. In order to be a friend, spouse, parent, or lover, you must be able to set aside the interpretive stance—the sometimes aloof and distant perspective of the "observer"—and enter into relationships with genuineness. You must also set aside the travails of conducting psychotherapy. Those working with patients suffering from severe psychopathology, in particular, struggle to leave it at the office, although their patients remain imprinted in their memories and may even intrude into their personal lives through emergencies and patient-initiated contacts outside of the session. Thus, it is probably not realistic to speak of always "leaving it at the office." Instead, it is more realistic to set boundaries and to modulate the intensity of therapist response to such work (Kaslow & Farber, 1995). A thoughtful attempt to define yourself outside of the office, therefore, entails creating boundaries and establishing a meaningful life sufficiently separate and rewarding to be a viable alternative to clinical work.

For many of us, this is easier said than done. Most of us admit that we are prone to overextension of work, and we need to make conscious efforts to construct boundaries to help us help our patients. To some extent, this is the price of socially defined success in our culture, but to some extent it also reflects some clinicians' characterological vulnerabilities. Those suffering from the central character trait of the selfless caretaker (Barbanelli, 1986) minimize their emotional needs in deference to the needs of others. As discussed in Chapter 2, some psychotherapists "need" to be needed. The approval-seeking preoccupation with recognition from significant others and suppression of anger are typically manifest. Always giving, but in the end, they typically feel deprived, isolated, underappreciated, and lacking a meaningful life outside of the office.

Significantly, the work-related distress of psychotherapists is not necessarily related to the number of their client contact hours (e.g., Firth-Cozens, 1992; Kramen-Kahn & Hansen, 1998; Sherman & Thelen, 1998). Thus, the common suggestion to cut back on the number of clients or reduce patient contact is not a panacea. Instead, one needs to selectively cut back and diversify one's activities by doing other things.

Subsequent chapters in this book traverse the variety of healthy escapes and creative activities outside of the consultation office available to the psychotherapist. All activities create stimulation, variety, and fresh challenges. Teaching, supervising, consulting at nearby agencies, conducting research, writing articles and books, or working in entirely different settings—all allow practitioners to define themselves as someone other than simply a psychotherapist. This same outcome can also be accomplished by pursuing parallel career interests outside the field, related or totally unrelated to psychotherapy.

Creating a broader definition of who you are as a professional can enable you to perceive yourself as more than a psychotherapist. Many colleagues acknowledge that doing so makes it easier to set aside the role when they leave the office (Guy, 1987). In fact, several of our master clinicians enthusiastically shared the value of pursuing other interests and activities, including teaching, research, media appearances, and writing. Out of our list of 19 self-care strategies, pursuing interests outside the consulting office ranked as the fifth most important. Clearly, many of the happiest and most successful psychotherapists have found that it is best to define themselves professionally rather broadly by pursuing a host of roles in addition to that of psychotherapist. One master clinician related the following during an interview:

> "Other professional activities help alleviate the stress of my practice. They take me one step back from the therapy process, and I can then see the big picture without getting lost in the details. It's also nice to function as a professional without feeling the pressure to do something about an urgent problem. I find that this helps to clarify my thoughts and provides a more relaxed opportunity for me to be creative."

In order for you to successfully set aside the role of the psychotherapist, your personal life must have meaning and joy outside of the healer role. Give careful consideration to your investment in pursuits that are independent of your work as a psychotherapist.

Clients outside the Office

Earlier, we discussed the need to carefully define the relationship between the client and therapist within the psychotherapy encounter. The focus then was primarily on the contacts that would occur within the context of the consulting office. We now consider contacts between client and therapist that might occur *outside* the office.

A concrete start is to demarcate work from home by developing a transition or decompression ritual. It convincingly marks the transition from work to nonwork. Representative rituals include sitting quietly for a minute before leaving for the day, saying a brief prayer, listening to relaxing music on the way home, spending some time alone reading, meditating for several minutes, changing clothes, and exercising (Mahoney, 2003; Neumann & Gamble, 1995). Something to formalize the physical and emotional transition.

Most ethics codes explicitly acknowledge that not all multiple relationships are unethical; however, multiple relationships that would reasonably be expected to cause impairment or risk exploitation or harm are deemed unethical (e.g., American Psychological Association, 2002). The intent is to strike a fair balance between benign and potentially therapeutic dual relationships, on the one hand, and blatantly exploitative relationships, on the other hand. The ethical line is that psychotherapists refrain from entering into a multiple relationship if it could reasonably be expected to impair the psychotherapist's objectivity, competence, or effectiveness in performing her function. The exact line here is murky and mired in professional controversy (see, e.g., Epstein, 1994, and Lazarus & Zur, 2002), but the essential point is that most dual relationships must be avoided in order to protect the client and the integrity of the treatment relationship.

Concretely, this means that the client and therapist will not pursue a relationship beyond the professional one already established. They will not meet together for other purposes, such as friendship, business, or romance. Having agreed upon this fact, there are still matters to discuss. Can the client call the therapist at home? Can she appear there for assistance? Will she meet individuals from the psychotherapist's personal life, such as a spouse, children, or friends? If the therapist and client should meet inadvertently outside of the office, should they acknowledge each other and visit together (Sharkin & Birky, 1992)? To what extent will the client have access to the personal life and relationships of the psychotherapist? These and similar concerns need to be discussed within the therapy relationship, keeping in mind the priority that is of paramount importance, namely, protecting the integrity of the psychotherapy relationship (Fremont & Anderson, 1988).

Interestingly, some clinicians experience difficulty in maintaining appropriate boundaries. They may be tempted to cross the boundaries themselves by making unnecessary phone calls to clients, sending letters or notes that are only vaguely related to the therapeutic work, or arranging to meet outside of the office for supposedly "psychotherapeutic" reasons. These behaviors can blur the roles and boundaries, with detrimental consequences for both the client's treatment and the private life of the psychotherapist.

Of course, more times than not, patients initiate the multiple relationships outside of the office. For patients with mild or solely Axis I disorders, gentle but firm reminders about the treatment contract will suffice to stop future contacts. But for patients with severe and Axis II disorders, more persistent efforts may be required.

One of our studies focused on protective measures taken by psychotherapists to ensure their safety and that of their loved ones (Guy et al., 1992). The top five measures were to decline to treat certain clients; refuse to disclose personal data to patients; prohibit clients from appearing at your home; locate the consultation office in a safe building; and specify intolerable patient behaviors. Other measures, as needed, should also be considered: avoid working alone in the office, install an office alarm system, obtain training in handling assaultive patients, and so on. The objective is to protect yourself and your life outside of the office.

Colleagues outside the Office

The practice of psychotherapy can easily absorb the entire life of the practitioner. It is a job—but much more than a job. Some psychotherapists prefer to "live" the job without interruption. In effect, they lose themselves in the persona of the psychotherapist or hide themselves in their patients' lives. They are always "on duty."

These individuals blur their life outside the office with their professional work. Social events typically center around conventions, workshops, retreats, supervision groups, and book discussion groups that focus on psychotherapy. Gatherings become meetings rather than parties. Colleagues become the primary, if not the only, friends of the practitioner. This blending of worlds is complete when the psychotherapist never has to stop being the clinician.

Although an exaggeration, this characterization is frighteningly too close for comfort. Consider whether colleagues in the profession have become the primary players, or even sole participants, in your private life outside the office. It will be extremely difficult to alleviate the distress of this profession, or maintain a balanced life, if there is no escape from professional colleagues who have become your only friends.

IN CLOSING

At the beginning of this chapter one of our workshop participants captured the essence of the dialectic between therapist self-care and clinical responsibilities. "How can I cut my hours down to 40 and walk away feeling justified? . . . Can I say 'no,' 'enough,' 'good enough for now' and still feel professional, effective, and ethical?" The incontrovertible answer is *Yes!*, but it takes considerable work to establish and maintain that delicate balance.

We advocate a mature synthesis to the dialectic of selfishness versus responsibility (Gilligan, 1982). Namely, define yourself, acknowledge your limitations, take control of your life, balance competing demands, and take an active stance toward your choices. In two words: "set boundaries."

The observation that therapists do not necessarily practice what they preach also applies to boundaries. One therapist (Penzer, 1984, p. 52) whimsically observed:

> We [psychotherapists] seem to possess our own unique brand of craziness seemingly endemic to and epidemic in our profession. Although not clearly identified in DSM-III, our dysfunction involves the promotion of wellness philosophies, goals and strategies, while imbibing homemade anti-wellness potions.

Top among the potions are short-lived boundary commitments, such as "I'm only going to work two nights a week," which have as little chance of implementation as a New Year's resolution. Like the diabetic physician who repeatedly fails to take her insulin, many of us fail to implement our own boundary advice. Some observers (e.g., Gladding, 1991) go so far as to label these boundary problems as therapist "self-abuse." Examples are practitioners who schedule too many clients in one day or who let clients consistently run over the allotted session time.

The probability of therapist impairment, particularly as it relates to client exploitation, is decreased by the clarification and strengthening of therapist boundaries (Skorupa & Agresti, 1993). The clinician who understands her role, and that of the client, will make better decisions regarding contacts both in and outside of the office. She will be better able to resist compromising the treatment relationship by encouraging other agendas, such as profit, companionship, or romance. Close relationships with family and friends assist the psychotherapist in confronting any growing tendencies toward substance abuse, suicidal behavior, or mental disorder. Honest scrutiny is more likely to occur within caring relationships with loved ones than within the work environment, where clients and colleagues have a wide variety of motives that make total disclosure difficult or unwise.

Our ardent hope in this chapter has been to canvass the multifarious manifestations of boundaries in and outside the office in a manner that informs, fuels, and guides your own self-care. Such boundary work takes considerable energy and deliberate commitment on your part. And it will entail careful attention to the nature of your relationships inside the office—with patients, colleagues, staff, and family—as well as outside the office with those same groups of people. Realistic boundaries are assuredly one key to successfully leaving it at the office.

SELF-CARE CHECKLIST

✓ Begin by understanding concretely your roles, responsibilities, and limitations as a psychotherapist; only then can you communicate and establish these boundaries with patients.

✓ Work under capacity (90%) so that emergencies, family demands, and self-care can be routinely accommodated.

✓ Be explicit with your clients about your professional expectations and limitations. Setting boundaries emerges in our research as the most frequent self-care strategy of mental health professionals.

✓ Secure goal consensus in a collaborative manner with patients early on in treatment to avoid subsequent boundary misunderstandings and confusion.

✓ Clearly delineate your policies regarding extra sessions, late appointments, extrasession telephone contacts, payment for services, and the like.

✓ Consider adopting an informed consent form as a written treatment contract.

✓ Establish a monitoring method to determine when a particular boundary has been crossed.

✓ Cultivate shared responsibility with patients for the change process and treatment outcome; avoid taking sole responsibility for psychotherapy.

✓ Craft your own professional bill of rights. What are your inalienable rights as a psychotherapist?

✓ Demand a livable wage and a "good enough" income.

✓ Set caseload boundaries: maintain your caseload at an effective number for you and limit the number of at-risk patients at any one time.

✓ Minimize as possible your out-of-session exposure to emergencies and patient incursions into your personal time.

✓ Take protective measures to ensure your physical safety and that of your loved ones. Decline to treat certain clients, refuse to disclose personal data, prohibit clients from appearing uninvited at your home, and make your office secure.

✓ Customize treatment to individual patients, but limit your bending. Determine whether you are bending too far.

✓ Learn to say "no" to clients, referral sources, agencies, and administrators; become a responsible assertive therapist.

✓ Rebuff inappropriate incursions into your practice by managed care organizations and other entities that would compromise your integrity and ethics.

✓ Delegate nonclinical work to staff or external services; focus on doing what you uniquely are trained and interested in doing.

✓ Be clear about posttermination contacts with clients. Saying good-bye to clients properly requires explicit statements concerning how, when, and why treatment may resume in the future.

✓ Beware of avarice. Are you working long hours out of financial necessity or because you are getting greedy?

✓ Bridge the gap between work hours and your loved ones by building in phone calls, personal visits, and short breaks.

✓ Demarcate the transition from work to nonwork with regular rituals, such as music, exercise, change of clothes, or meditation.

✓ Transfer difficult patients—for an evaluation, a second opinion, or for treatment elsewhere—from a position of strength.

✓ Remember that your clients are not there to meet your needs; treatment relationships are not reciprocal.

✓ Define your relationships with colleagues with care. Transference influences these relationships, too.

✓ Let your hair down with family and friends. They want you to be genuine, spontaneous, and unprofessional.

✓ Establish an identity and life apart from your psychotherapist role. Don't get stale!

✓ Zealously protect your personal time with family and friends; work is work and home is home.

✓ Avoid friendships exclusively with clinical colleagues, as social gatherings with them may quickly deteriorate into work meetings.

✓ Embrace a mature synthesis of the dialectic between commitment to self and commitment to patients. It is possible to balance both through realistic boundaries.

RECOMMENDED READING

Epstein, R. S. (1994). *Keeping boundaries: Maintaining safety and integrity in the psychotherapeutic process.* Washington, DC: American Psychiatric Press.

Johnston, S. H., & Farber, B. A. (1996). The maintenance of boundaries in psychotherapeutic practice. *Psychotherapy, 33,* 391–402.

Knapp, S., & Slattery, J. M. (2004). Professional boundaries in nontraditional settings. *Professional Psychology: Research and Practice, 35,* 553–558.

Pope, K. S., Sonne, J. L., & Holroyd, J. (1993). *Sexual feelings in psychotherapy.* Washington, DC: American Psychological Association.

CHAPTER 7

Restructuring Cognitions

with Maria A. Turkson

Cognitive restructuring for psychotherapists is steeped in ironies. Although intellectually aware of the irrational beliefs explored in rational-emotive therapy and the depressogenic assumptions of cognitive therapy, we therapists all fall prey to these cognitive errors. A predilection for dispassionate examination does not immunize us to the perils of the secular world. We are blissfully human, and, as such, we are subject to the same corrosive logic as our fellow humans.

Indeed, the father of cognitive-behavioral therapy, Albert Ellis, writes (1987, p. 364) that irrationalities "persist among highly intelligent, educated, and relatively little disturbed individuals" and "seem to flow from deep-seated and almost ineradicable human tendencies toward fallibility, overgeneralization, wishful thinking, gullibility, and short-range hedonism." Assuming too much responsibility for our patients, catastrophizing over a case, and thinking dichotomously about the outcome of psychotherapy plague us all at times. Ironically, we engage in the very dysfunctional thoughts that we desperately teach our clients to avoid.

It's hard to be dispassionate about a subject when it's yourself. Nonetheless, identifying and challenging our faulty assumptions are keys to therapist self-care. This chapter focuses on cognitive restructuring: identifying and challenging problematic thinking that serves to maintain negative feelings and self-defeating behavior. We explore and consider the remediation of prevalent "musturbations" (Ellis, 1984) and cognitive errors (Beck, Rush, Shaw, & Emery, 1979) that psychotherapists inflict upon themselves. In a significant way, this entire volume is devoted to remediating the cognitive errors of psychotherapists; however, in this chapter we focus on specific examples and methods of cognitive restructuring.

We employ the cognitive-behavioral term of *cognitive restructuring* in this chapter, but intend it in a transtheoretical manner. We use it as a broad process across theoretical orientations rather than a specific cognitive-behavioral method. Cognitive therapists are not the first or only ones to identify perfectionist strivings and cognitive errors. Psychoanalysts, in particular, have written extensively about the persistence of unrealistic and unrealizable analytic ideals of patient outcomes and therapist methods. One author (Abend, 1986, p. 566) reminds us that, although experience certainly dictates that perfectionist goals are all but impossible to attain, they continue nevertheless to influence both theory and aspirations. Most therapists try to live up to the inflated ideals of the masters, from Freud on down.

Solution-focused therapy, too, reminds us to reauthor our own narratives. Consider these examples of cognitive restructuring via rewriting our stories about clients (based on Clifton, Doan, & Mitchell, 1990):

- If instead of being viewed as resistant, this client were viewed as being scared, how would my story about her change?
- If I were more sensitive to the predicaments of my clients, and less wed to a therapy model, what might I notice that has gone unseen before?
- If I assumed that the patient had coping resources and was responsible for her own life, how would I think differently about her? About my own burden and role as a therapist?
- Which do you think is most in charge of your professional life at present: a hero/heroine role or a victim role?

Solution-focused therapy underscores the difference between the therapist's approach to a session with a "problem" versus a "solution" mindset. Just as clients often become "stuck" in their emotional experience, therapists can become mired in their negative reactions to clients or fixated on labeling the client's problematic way of being (e.g., resistance, intellectualization, transference). This change to "solutions" can empower therapists by focusing on what is controllable and changeable (i.e., themselves!).

Similarly, humanistic therapists remind us to "cognitively restructure" our reactions to clients via empathy. When sitting with a client who criticizes your skills as a therapist, or projects anger toward you because she is not "getting better," you can grasp those responses from an empathic place (e.g., "The client is experiencing a great deal of pain"). It is more difficult to feel anger when you hear her message as one of helplessness and pain rather than filtering the message through your own experience (e.g., "I'm annoyed that the client is calling me a lousy therapist," or "The nerve of her to become angry at me when I'm working so hard!").

In our interviews preparing for this book, one of our master clinicians bluntly stated:

> "Stress is always self-created. Stress means that it is difficult, and when you do not have cognitive restructuring you define the difficulty as awful, horrible, that it shouldn't exist. When you do cognitive restructuring, then you define it as a pain in the ass, period, and you don't get depressed about it. For example, when the clients are a pain in the ass then you define it as a pain in the ass, instead of horrible and awful."

By heeding this candid redefinition of stress, you can transform, in Freud's terms, neurotic misery into ordinary annoyance.

SELF-MONITORING

Cognitive restructuring starts with self-awareness and self-monitoring. We begin by recognizing what we tell ourselves, explicitly or implicitly, regarding our performance and identity as psychotherapists. A few minutes of thoughtful reflection, collecting data to test our assumptions, concerned sharing with significant others—all of these alert us to the self-deceptions that creep into our thinking and eventually into our practice.

As therapists, our introspective skills allow us to monitor internal dialogue. For example, a client relates an experience in session, and you cannot conjure up a compelling or accurate empathic reflection. You demean yourself: "Why can't I feel or resonate today?" After a few moments your self-monitoring may recognize this instance of faulty logic. There is no singular interpretation or reflection, and even if there was, there is no reason to expect perfection in each clinical transaction. Or perhaps there is no need to analyze or comment at that moment!

Self-monitoring permits us to recognize our cognitive errors, determine our faulty assumptions, and prescribe an alternative. If our irrational thinking is not immediately apparent to us, it very likely will stick out (like a neon light in the darkness) to others, especially our coworkers. All for the better! Another therapist's viewpoint may provide a new spin on our thinking. One of our clinical colleagues, for example, artfully points out our heavy sighing between sessions, a guaranteed tip-off that our perfectionistic expectations are getting the best of us that day. A little collegial prompting begets self-monitoring and disputations.

We consider self-monitoring internal dialogue to be the indispensable first step in battling our cognitive errors. Awareness alone, of course, is insufficient in combating the therapist "musturbations" and shoulds. Intellectual insight by itself, as Freud reminded us, is about as efficacious as providing a starving person with only a dinner menu. But awareness and insight begin the process of cognitive restructuring.

FIVE THERAPIST MUSTURBATIONS

"What do I do to keep from obsessing about a woman whose husband has just speculated on what knife he would use to kill her; a borderline patient who is chewing me out for not immediately returning her nonemergency phone call; or a staff member who has neglected to arrange for a repair, resulting in the ceiling falling in during a rainstorm?" So begins rational-emotive therapist Janet Wolfe's (2000, p. 581) "A Vacation from Musturbation," an article appearing in the Self-Care Corner in *Professional Psychology*, which one of us (JCN) coedited a few years ago. Her answer: "I try as much as possible to practice what I preach during the work hours and to take my philosophy with me when I leave the office."

Over the years Albert Ellis (1984) has gathered the common irrationalities or lies we psychotherapists tell ourselves. His list of five "musturbations"—things that therapists tell themselves they must do— includes several, corollary irrationalities. The following are extracted from his "How to Deal with Your Most Difficult Client—You."

Musturbation 1: I Must Be Successful with My Patients, Practically All of the Time

The corollary musturbations include (1) I must always make brilliant interpretations or empathic responses, (2) I must help my clients *more*, and (3) I must not fail with any of my clients, but if I do, it is my fault and I'm a lousy person! After our putting in years of graduate training and after our best empathic efforts, some patients have the audacity to get worse. Shouldn't they have the common courtesy of getting better?!

The reality of psychotherapy, of course, is that success is neither automatic nor universal. Any therapist who assumes she has to succeed every time will eventually find great disappointment. We will not be successful with every client for multiple reasons; to say that you *must* always do so is completely contrary to the definition of being human.

We are reminded here of a particular case, involving a schizophrenic woman, that personally affected Carl Rogers enough to impair his own functioning as a therapist and as a human being. This case is an example of how psychotherapists, believing success will come with every patient, can mistakenly ignore their own problems for the sake of their client. Before treating the woman, Rogers "had come to understand the importance of the *client's* feelings in the relationship, [but] his own personal background [suppressing feelings as a child] still held him back from giving due attention to the therapist's feelings" (Kirschenbaum, 1979, p. 191). Difficulties began when Rogers, the paragon of empathy, substituted apathy for his traditional warmth whenever the woman's disturbance and dependence threatened him.

Although not succeeding with the patient, Rogers continued treatment. In his own words, "I started to feel it was a real drain on me, yet I stubbornly felt that I *should* be able to help her and permitted the contacts to continue long after they had ceased to be therapeutic, and it involved only suffering for me." Moreover, recognizing "that many of her insights were sounder" than his, Rogers lost confidence in himself. Although Rogers suffered deep distress as a result of this experience, he worked through it and eventually liked himself more. Even the most eminent therapists, like the rest of us mortals, are often blindsided by impossible expectations.

What are adaptive alternative cognitions? That psychotherapy succeeds with most, but not all, patients. That we are human and will make errors. Yes, it would be highly preferable to always make brilliant interpretations and always have good judgments, but that is unrealistic and unobtainable.

Musturbation 2: I Must Be One of the World's Most Outstanding Therapists

Two corollary musturbations are that "every therapy session with clients (including difficult clients) must be good" and "I must be an eminent therapist."

In a self-care symposium we organized a few years back, Judy Beck (1997) spoke movingly of her travails when comparing her clinical and scholarly performance to her father, Aaron T. Beck, one of the founders of cognitive therapy. She was bound to feel inferior, as we all would, given the impossible standards. It is a constant struggle to make realistic comparisons instead of perfectionist evaluations. Judy Beck advises us to compare ourselves to same-aged peers in similar circumstances.

As Ellis ardently puts it in "How I Manage to Be a 'Rational' Rational Emotive Behavior Therapist" (1995, p. 4):

> There is no damned—or undamned—reason why I *absolutely must* be an outstanding therapist, colleague, socialite or anything else! I am determined to always give myself unconditional self-acceptance (USA) whether or not I perform well and whether or not I am loved and approved.

The resultant internal dialogue might be "I would like to be an outstanding therapist and have good sessions with all clients; but if I cannot, I *can* still be a competent therapist and enjoy doing therapy." Moreover, "Why do I *have* to be a well-known therapist? Am I afraid that if I do not work so ardently and compulsively, that I might not be a good therapist?" We don't have to be labeled as "the best" to perform well. If in the process of establishing a distinguished career we succeed in making ourselves disturbed with our own stringent, absolutistic views, haven't we sacrificed too much?

Musturbation 3: I Must Be Liked and Respected by All My Clients

Several related fallacies frequently follow: I must like all my clients, but if I do not, I must not allow myself to have negative feelings toward them; I must not insist my clients work too hard in therapy; and I must avoid sensitive issues that might disturb or upset my clients.

Many of us erroneously conclude that a patient's liking us is equivalent to good psychotherapy. Yet, gentle confrontation is the other side of caring. We need to be caring, but we also need to be tough (Whitaker & Bumberry, 1988). The therapeutic relationship parallels good parenting. Just as a good parent provides a child with nurturance and discipline, to help a patient grow you provide support and honestly address problem areas.

Ideally, conducting psychotherapy should be pleasant. However, unpleasantness is sometimes a reality, a part of the vicissitudes of life. Asking patients to address difficult topics, pushing them to work harder, and recommending that they expose themselves to previously avoided situations will make the pathway to healing bumpy. During these potentially stressful times, patients may retaliate by becoming angry, canceling sessions, or even changing therapists. Just because you are a helper doesn't mean the transactions between you and your client will always feel comfortable.

Musturbation 4: Since I Am a Hard-Working Therapist, My Clients Should Be Equally Persevering

Corollary musturbations concerning the anticipation of cooperative patients include: (1) My clients should be tractable, not impossible! (2) My clients should always have their homework assignments done on time; and (3) I should only have YAVIS (young, attractive, verbal, intelligent, and successful) clients! Don't hard-working, successful therapists deserve hardworking, successful patients?

Is there a healthier alternative? Perhaps. "It would be ideal if all my clients were hard-working, but if they aren't, I will still accept and try to help them despite their imperfections." We all feel occasionally frustrated by our patients' lack of motivation and further nettled by their apparent unconcern or lackadaisical attitude. This comes with the job description. Your client is paying you to do your job—who says she must do hers? You? For a therapist, detached compassion is sometimes the way of survival. We can pitch the benefits of change, but we can't make the client buy it.

Musturbation 5: I Must Be Able to Enjoy Myself during Therapy

Corollary thoughts might be (1) I must use therapeutic techniques that I enjoy regardless of their benefit to the client; (2) I must use only simple techniques that will not drain my energy; and (3) my sessions can be used to solve my own problems as well as the client's problems. These thoughts converge on the entitlement or grandiosity afflicting some psychotherapists after many years of practice.

Creeping entitlement can be met with cognitive restructuring. "I would be overjoyed if my therapy sessions helped me to solve some of my own problems; however, my job is to help my clients, not me." Work is called work for a reason. It's not necessarily fun, exciting, or simple, but it is often arduous.

To mentally combat the hassles at work, Ellis (1995, p. 4) recommends his musturbatory-busting rationale:

> The conditions that often prevail in therapy don't *have to be* always easy, comfortable, and enjoyable. In fact, they often aren't. Unfortunate! Inconvenient! But not the end of the world. Just a royal pain in the ass! Now how can I do my best to improve them—or *unwhiningly accept* what I can't change? What's my alternative? More silly whining!

As every half-conscious psychotherapist knows, awareness alone is insufficient in rectifying such musturbations and shoulds. Instead, irrational beliefs are often deep-seated—tenaciously implanted at the core of our personality—and require vigilance in identifying and disputing them. Just as we do in our clinical work. We alleviate our emotional distress only by *practicing* rational beliefs, *practicing* appropriate emotions (such as annoyance instead of misery), and *practicing* desirable behaviors.

COGNITIVE ERRORS

Experienced therapists benefit from many of the same cognitive therapy methods as their patients (Beck, 1997). For example, monitoring one's overly busy schedule and rating pleasure and mastery of activities can help the therapist discover what changes need to be made. Or, for another example, uncovering one's expectations of self and others and assessing the advantages and disadvantages for holding such standards can lead to a more functional reassessment. Recognition and modification of a dysfunctional comparison set—such as Judy Beck's earlier example of comparing herself to higher achieving mentors instead of similarly situated peers—often improves self-confidence.

Following are a medley of cognitive errors frequently committed by psychotherapists and a compilation of potential cognitive solutions.

Selective Abstraction

A patient in psychotherapy with you for 3 months is not getting better. You tell yourself you've done everything possible thus far. You listened attentively and resonated with the patient's experience. You conducted treatment in accord with the research evidence. You tried several treatment approaches. You have prescribed (or referred for) psychotropic medication. Nothing seems to work. Yet, twinges of guilt and doubt pass through your mind: "I'm a failure as a therapist!" and "I should have listened to my mother and become a lawyer!" Several other failure cases from the past invade your consciousness. Suddenly you are feeling worthless and inept; to compound your self-doubts, you realize that your patient is the one who's suffering the most here, and maybe, just maybe, it's your fault.

Sound familiar? We are so accustomed to perfection. Our work means so much to us: We've devoted a substantial part of our lives educating ourselves for the work. And to get this far in the profession we needed excellent grades and work habits—not average, but excellent.

The point is this: we are accustomed to being competent and successful. "The absolutely perfect practitioner is, of course, a misguided and misguiding illusion, but it still operates in the tacit life ordering that goes on in psychotherapists' lives" (Mahoney, 1991, p. 352) Expecting perfection in practice contributes to our own mental suffering.

We can be like Winnicott's (1958) good-enough mother. Even when we make mistakes in therapy or disappoint the client in some way, we can process these empathic failures. It's not the end of the world. For example, one of us was on vacation when a client was going through a particularly difficult time. The next postvacation session provided what Winnicott describes as an opportunity to reexperience the failure situation. Acknowledging that the client felt abandoned furthered the work of therapy and increased the relational bond.

Selective abstraction, as you may recall, is the mistake of believing that the only events that matter are failures and that you should measure yourself by errors (Beck et al., 1979). You probably also recall several ways to minimize selective abstraction: track your experiences to determine successes and failures; accept the inevitable limitations of your therapeutic skills; and distinguish between case failures and yourself as a failure. More simply, rejoice in your successes, accept your human limitations, and offer yourself unconditional acceptance. Just because you have fail*ed* doesn't mean you are a fail*ure*.

Consider the exemplar of negative outcomes in psychotherapy. Approximately 5–15% of patients will experience increased distress and deterioration while in psychotherapy (not necessarily as a result of psychotherapy). We conveniently forget the 75%+ who are successes and preoccupy ourselves with the failures. This is not to suggest, of course, that we should dismiss the failures as inconvenient artifacts; rather, it is to suggest a psychological re-equilibrium. We recommend that you track or "log" your success experiences.

Once they are tracked, remember those successes. As we recommended in Chapter 3, whenever you begin obsessing about a recent difficulty or failure, remind yourself of the scores of successful cases in which you have genuinely assisted people. Savor your successes and acknowledge your contributions to bettering the human condition.

We can also measure success differently than complete remission of symptoms and total patient satisfaction (Edelwich & Brodsky, 1980). We can focus on the process and our efforts rather than solely on the results, set more modest or achievable goals for patients, and not expect immediate results. And, as we have emphasized, focus on the successes and not just the failures.

In the movie *It's a Wonderful Life*, the guardian angel Clarence tried to comfort George Bailey, who was dissatisfied with what seemed like a failure-filled life. Clarence said, "You just don't know how much you've done." We must be our own "Clarence" and force ourselves to see all the good we have accomplished. While we cannot turn back time and observe our patients' lives without our help, we *can* imagine it. There surely are many cases where our clients' lives were significantly improved through our presence and intervention.

Overwhelming Tasks

Just as patients may be distressed because they take on more work or responsibility than is expected of them, psychotherapists are susceptible to the same mistakes. We can fall prey to a messianic complex and take on too many patients, too many projects, or too many particularly disturbed clients. As we know from cognitive therapy (Beck et al., 1979, p. 188), our impression of the world must be reconceptualized from "it is overwhelming" to (1) "What are the specific problems?" and (2) "What are the specific solutions?" The motto might be: Define and solve in an orderly rational way.

You might counter that real-world problems are not so easily opera-tionalized nor solutions so evident. You could protest, "John and Jim, I am working in an overwhelming, understaffed public agency" or "I simply cannot do less or make less money." That may well be, but we can break large, vague problems down into workable parts that can be more easily solved. If this sounds like advice you frequently give your patients, it prob-ably is.

For starters, we are probably accomplishing more than we realize. By recording our actions in a log or diary, the record will show that we are accomplishing something. Cognitive therapists wisely maintain that tak-ing some action represents a partial success. The cognitive distortion rep-resented in the statement "The task is so problematic it cannot be done" is corrected.

The cognitive model of distress further holds that many people take on more work than they need to. For example, therapists typically think "I must see at least seven patients every day" or "I must allow at least 50 min-utes for a session." Still others wrongly think they are expected to do more than they need to. For example, "I must practice full-time and teach a course at night plus be a great parent." Folks who think this rigidly, according to cognitive theory, actually *believe* they cannot withdraw from any of their endeavors.

For people to obtain a realistic view of their workload and others' expectations, Beck and other cognitive therapists suggest disputing unre-alistic expectations, constructing boundaries, and assertively protecting those boundaries. For instance, "My private practice and children assume priority. Thus, I will continue the practice and be a good parent. However, there is no law stating that I *have* to teach in the evening."

In our own lives, we periodically enter a "just say no" stage. Say "no" to new patients, say "no" to writing offers, say "no" to additional work-shops. Of course, we must then cognitively tackle the emotional effects of saying "no": the mild guilt in disappointing people, the potential regret in not making extra money, the nagging doubt that we may not have similar opportunities in the future. We have found cognitive restructuring to be effective in reducing the emotional effects during such moments.

Assuming Causality

Psychotherapists often incorrectly assign the blame or responsibility for adverse events to themselves—assuming personal causality. The mis-guided, self-referencing belief is that we are to blame for all misfortune. If a client succeeds in therapy, it's her responsibility; if a client fails in ther-apy, it's our responsibility (fault). Attributing most adverse occurrences to a personal deficiency, such as a lack of ability or effort, is assuming per-sonal causality.

As we write this chapter, hundreds of subscribers to the e-mail network of the Society of Clinical Psychology were mistakenly removed because of a hardware error. Dozens of these doctorally trained psychologists posted their belief that they were omitted from the subscription list because they thought they had annoyed the list manager or had committed a grievous insult. They were, in short, assuming personal causality for a random technical error.

In medicine, physicians are trained early and well to realize that some patients, such as those in end-state terminal cancer, will probably never improve; but they try to help nonetheless. In psychotherapy, we intellectually acknowledge these constraints but have not yet learned to accept our limits openly.

One of us (JCN) painfully recalls conducting therapy with a couple who decided amicably to get divorced. I took it hard until my wife reminded me, in simple and caring words, that I did not create the relationship difficulties. This simple observation exploded my largely unconscious belief that somehow I was responsible for reversing time—like Superman circling the planet Earth to turn back the clock—and for fixing their extensive problems. We all struggle not to feel responsible for solving and eradicating our clients' problems, however vexing and long-standing.

The weight of self-reproach can be lifted and some objectivity gained through the disattribution technique (Beck et al., 1979, p. 158). The disattribution technique is a simple yet powerful method. It entails recognizing that you impose excessively stringent standards on yourself and disputing the belief that you are entirely responsible for negative events.

Consider the case of Dr. G, a conscientious and scrupulous practitioner who entered personal therapy with one of us because she felt responsible for the suicide of a 27-year-old patient. Some of her self-blaming statements were: "If my schedule wasn't so booked, I could have seen her more often" and "I should have been more observant during that last session—I could've noticed some sign of her self-destructive intent." After several sessions and grief work, Dr. G related that she had actually taken considerable care with this difficult patient: she had revamped her schedule to accommodate additional sessions, carefully monitored the patient's medications, sought the counsel of the patient's two previous therapists who also had little success, and had taken other measures to safeguard herself and her quite disturbed patient. After applying the disattribution technique, Dr. G gradually realized that not only did she conduct "good-enough" psychotherapy but she also went beyond her customary duty. Finally, Dr. G recognized that she was not responsible for this woman's death. Neurotic guilt gave way to understandable loss and pain—a tragically common occupational hazard of working with severely disturbed humans.

In addition to assuming personal causality—"I am responsible for these bad things"—psychotherapists often assume temporal causality—"Bad things happened in the past, so they will happen in the future." Consider these negative prophetic statements: "My last two long-term cases never improved, so this one probably won't either"; and "Another depressed person. Therapy will now be difficult because it's hard to change the negative thinking. This process is draining and monotonous. Therefore I won't be doing my best therapy." How do we know these predictions are true? We don't.

When you catch yourself making doom-and-gloom statements, you may profit by carefully analyzing your assumptions. Making them explicit, writing them down, or sharing your arguments with a colleague may sound ridiculous. You will probably protest initially: "For heaven's sake! I'm a therapist, I don't need to express my thoughts in writing—surely I'm more sophisticated than that! And share my irrational thoughts with colleagues? They'll think I'm an idiot!" This resistance frequently betrays another belief commonplace among self-sufficient therapists: the fear of appearing incompetent. Taking a few moments to contemplate your internal talk, what you have written, or a colleague's comments may bring to light your own overly pessimistic reasoning.

Also, instead of treating past events as totally predictive, you can list other factors influencing the outcome. For example, there are a number of patient and environmental variables that have an impact on the outcome of psychotherapy. Two patient characteristics that predict slow or little success are high functional impairment and low readiness to change (see Norcross, 2002). Perhaps the patient's environment, your clinical setting, or the available resources simply do not offer the number of sessions or intensity of services needed. Taking the time to identify other factors that may influence the outcome will eliminate using past experience as the sole predictor of future events.

Catastrophizing

Anticipating the worst outcome protects us: at least we won't be surprised when it happens. However, doomsday prophecy also contributes to therapist decay. At lunch the other day, one of our colleagues, a counselor employed at the local community mental health center (CMHC), acerbically insisted that "no one comes out of the partial hospitalization program better than when they came in." After empathizing with his difficulties in battling chronic disorders with severely underfunded resources, we gently chided him to reevaluate whether catastrophizing his program's outcomes did anything to improve the situation.

There are at least three salutary cognitive strategies for treating catastrophizing: (1) show that the worst *did* not actually happen ("Did that really occur?"), (2) determine the actual likelihood that the worst may happen ("What are the real probabilities?"), and (3) evaluate the consequences should the worst scenario improbably occur ("What would be the worst that could happen?"). With our frustrated CMHC colleague, respectful inquiries revealed that the worst did not actually happen—the partial hospitalization program surely does have successes. If the worst did occur for certain patients who deteriorated, then they were immediately referred to the inpatient unit, a real probability for many of these chronically and severely disturbed patients. When the worst did occur, the patients underwent a brief inpatient stay and then returned to the partial hospitalization program. While our colleague's emotional frustration in working with such a difficult population is readily understandable, his cognitive distortions unfortunately reinforced our collective susceptibility to negative thinking. We—all of us—are more human than otherwise.

Dichotomous Thinking

How many times have you said "I got nothing done today" or "All my sessions were tough"—or even "Managed care is destroying my private practice"? Dichotomous (either–or) thinking is both a cause and a result of psychotherapist distress. A related attribute of this dysfunctional mindset is viewing negative consequences as irreversible.

Evaluating events on a continuum is an effective antidote for dichotomous thinking. Speaking in quantitative terms may seem like a mechanical exercise, but it pays off. For example, instead of "I got nothing done today," perhaps "I accomplished a few minor tasks today and a small portion of a major task." Rather than "all my sessions were tough," perhaps "50% of my sessions were trying and 50% were moderate" would be a more accurate description of your day.

To modify extreme thinking and to view negative consequences as both reversible and only temporary, look for partial gains in reversals (Beck et al., 1979). What positive element can you find in a day that was otherwise "a complete disaster"? If you weren't performing well, perhaps you made some mistakes while conducting therapy. "My day was a total mess!" might be mentally transformed into "Now that I know what mistakes to avoid, I will conduct better therapy next time." In fact, these struggles *do* make us better psychotherapists. In *On Being a Psychotherapist*, Goldberg (1986, p. 109) maintains that if the practitioner regards her own struggles not as signs of weakness and shame, but as pangs of passion, caring, and concern, then the practitioner is more likely to offer clients a more meaningful therapeutic experience.

Dichotomous thinking is a fitting example of rigidity. To place all of your experiences into two groups (e.g., good or bad) is unrealistic. As we have seen, there are positives even in "bad" clinical situations.

MANAGING COUNTERTRANSFERENCE

A pervasive struggle for all psychotherapists is thinking "straight" about their countertransference, that is, those internal and external reactions in which unresolved conflicts (usually but not always unconscious) are implicated (Gelso & Hayes, 2002). How do we think through our client-induced rage or dysphoria or sexual arousal? Countertransference requires all of the self-care methods in our arsenal (and in this book), but a few words here on cognitive restructuring.

The nascent research on managing countertransference highlights five interrelated skills: self-insight, self-integration, empathy, anxiety management, and conceptualizing ability (Gelso & Hayes, 2002). Four of these five directly concern the cognitive operations of the therapist, whereas self-integration refers to the therapist's possession of an intact, basically healthy, character structure. These serve as a cognitive roadmap.

Self-insight refers to the extent to which the therapist is aware of her own feelings, including countertransference feelings, and understands their basis. Empathy permits the therapist to focus on the patient's needs despite difficulties she may be experiencing with the work and inclinations to attend to one's own needs. Also, empathic ability may be part of sensitivity to one's own feelings, including countertransference feelings, which in turn ought to prevent the acting out of countertransference. Anxiety management refers to the therapist allowing herself to experience anxiety but also possessing the internal skill to control and understand anxiety so that it does not bleed over into responses to patients. Finally, conceptualizing ability reflects the therapist's ability to draw on professional theory and to comprehend the patient's dynamics in relation to the therapeutic alliance.

All of these skills are brought to bear on understanding the patient's dynamics, your response to them, and then responding constructively despite your anxiety. When a patient screams at you, your awareness and interpretation of projective identification enable you not to scream back. When a patient argues incessantly with you, perhaps rekindling parental or sibling conflicts, your cognitive restructuring and anxiety management help you label it as enactment of old relational patterns, and you do not argue in return. Identifying, labeling, and managing your intense affective reactions all require advanced cognitive restructuring. These skills increase your capacity for affect regulation and demarcating the boundary between your emotional life and that of your patient. In this way, your cognitive self-care is crucial to remaining present, supportive, and effective with patients.

IN CLOSING

We end this chapter—perhaps we should have begun it—with the ultimate psychotherapist fallacy: "I should have no emotional problems. After all, I am a therapist!" We all chuckle appreciatively at this palpable nonsense—but also at the self-recognition that a small part of us secretly clings to it. Most psychotherapists suffer from idealized perfectionism and outrageous expectations; then, to top it off, they feel ashamed and guilty for acknowledging their perfectionistic expectations! Take comfort in Freud's (1937/1964, p. 247) early recognition that "analysts are people who have learned to practice a particular art; alongside of this, they may be allowed to be human beings like anyone else."

Yes, if therapists were not human, we'd be able to transcend dysfunctional thinking and avoid the occupational hazards. But the lament reflects, in itself, wishful thinking instead of cognitive restructuring. Just as industrial workers must undergo safety training in working with heavy machinery, therapists must practice cognitive restructuring as a sort of mental safety, self-maintenance routine.

While we are it, let us create realistic expectations of self-care. If they are not careful, some of our workshop participants transfer their perfectionism to their self-care. One of our participants wrote that the lasting lesson of the workshop for her was "To be more realistic about what's doable in a certain time period. I am not setting myself up for a feeling that I have failed." Please practice cognitive restructuring against unrealistic self-care expectations.

If only we took our advice more seriously! (Kottler, 1993). It is poignantly ironic that the skills we teach our patients seem like foreign concepts when we combat our own difficulties. It is easy to discern someone else's difficulties when you are an objective observer; it is hard to objectively observe yourself.

Assuming too much responsibility for our patients, catastrophizing over a case, and thinking dichotomously about the outcome of psychotherapy are just a few examples. Some empathic but persistent disputations help. Who is responsible for patients' psychopathology and decisions? How many cases are truly outstanding successes, on the one hand, or spectacular failures, on the other? Not many; it is always a continuum of outcomes.

Recognizing and managing our own musturbations, cognitive errors, and countertransference reactions are paramount to leaving it at the

office. If we can offer ourselves the same empathy and cognitive restructuring we strive to provide to our patients, then we will indeed count ourselves among the successful patients we have treated.

SELF-CARE CHECKLIST

✓ Self-monitor your internal dialogue regarding your performance and
your patients via thoughtful reflection, collecting data to dispute
cognitive errors, or sharing with significant others.

✓ Compare your clinical and scholarly performance to same-aged peers
in similar circumstances, not to authorities.

✓ Track your overly busy schedule and rate pleasure and mastery
of activities to help you discover what changes need to be
made.

✓ Self-treat the error of selective abstraction by determining actual
successes and failures, accepting the inevitable limitations of your
therapeutic skills, and distinguishing between case failures and yourself
as a failure.

✓ Think through the transferential feelings directed to you; to whom are
they aimed and to whom do they belong?

✓ Beware of absolutist thinking: musturbation ("I must be ... ") and the
tyranny of the shoulds ("I should have ... "). They can affect you as
much as your patients.

✓ Dispute the common fallacy that "good psychotherapy is equivalent to
having all patients like us."

✓ Recall that the other side of caring consists of confrontation. Caring
about others includes being honest and tough at times.

✓ Reassure yourself that the conditions in psychotherapy, as well as in
life, are not always easy. This is unfortunate but not catastrophic.

✓ Remind yourself that you cannot cure every patient and that some
patients will not succeed with you.

✓ Balance the amount of time you dwell on your successful cases and
your frustrating cases.

✓ Redefine success as a process rather than an end result. Success
includes your effort, and mini- or partial achievements, not simply the
complete remission of patient symptoms.

✓ Assertively reduce unrealistic demands made on you: don't take on
more work than you need to or wrongly believe you're expected to
do more.

✓ Recognize that your patients do not have to be as hard-working or persevering as you.

✓ Ask three critical questions—Did that really occur?, What are the probabilities?, and What is the worst that could happen?—when you catastrophize about you and your clients.

✓ Catch yourself when assuming blame (i.e., personal causality) for events in clients' lives and consider alternative explanations.

✓ Calculate real probabilities when thinking about treatment outcomes. The worst happens only infrequently—to you or to your patients.

✓ Evaluate treatment success on a continuum to avoid dichotomous thinking; psychotherapy outcomes rarely fall on either extreme of a continuum.

✓ Use self-insight, empathy, anxiety management, and conceptualizing ability when experiencing countertransference reactions.

✓ Confront the ultimate psychotherapist fallacy: "I should not have emotional problems. After all, I am a therapist!" Yes, you are an expert on human behavior—but you're still nutty at times!

✓ Create realistic expectations for your self-care; avoid perfectionist tendencies toward eradicating your perfectionism.

✓ Offer yourself unconditional self-acceptance (USA) as a psychotherapist and as a person.

RECOMMENDED READING

Beck, J. S., & Butler, A. C. (2005). Treating psychotherapists with cognitive therapy. In J. D. Geller, J. C. Norcross, & D. E. Orlinsky (Eds.), *The psychotherapist's own psychotherapy*. New York: Oxford University Press.

Ellis, A. (1984). How to deal with your most difficult client—you. *Psychotherapy in Private Practice, 2*, 25–35.

Wolfe, J. L. (2000). A vacation from musturbation. *Professional Psychology: Research and Practice, 31*, 581–583.

CHAPTER 8

Sustaining
Healthy Escapes

with Rhonda S. Karg

> True happiness, we are told, consists in getting out of one's
> self. But the point is not only to get out—you've got to stay
> out; and to stay out you must have some absorbing errand.
> —HENRY JAMES

Escapism is one of the most effective and popular methods of psychotherapist self-care. As part of our human nature, we clearly *want* to escape;
as part of our healing burden, we may even *need* to escape periodically to
minimize the corrosive effects of conducting psychotherapy. Occasional
escapes allow us to temporarily separate ourselves from our professional
identities and activities as we submerge our awareness in another experience. The common thread among the diverse escapes considered in this
chapter is occasional release from professional responsibilities and the
concomitant immersion in alternative outlets.

Escape can denote many behaviors. We are all familiar with the
unhealthy escapes or false cures—alcohol abuse, isolation, sexual acting
out, self-medication—that ultimately multiply the very sources of distress
that they were intended to ameliorate. Like healthy diversions, maladaptive escapism provides a source of gratification and relief but exacts a
cost—physically, psychologically, spiritually, and interpersonally. As we

have all repeatedly witnessed in our patients, unhealthy escape itself becomes a new burden.

In contrast to unhealthy avoidance, healthy escapes denote embracing balance and wellness. They encompass constructive behaviors that invoke and blend diversion, self-nurturance, and relaxation in ways that balance work with respite. Healthy escapism, as we mean it in this chapter, means taking breaks during our workday and leaving the office altogether, so that we may shortly return to our personal and professional lives with renewed energy and a fresh perspective. In this chapter, we explore healthy escapes in and outside the office, after a brief consideration of the dark side of unhealthy escapes.

UNHEALTHY ESCAPES

We psychotherapists, being more human than otherwise, are not immune to mistreating our distress. In fact, the research indicates that psychotherapists are at high risk for being seduced by the lures of unhealthy escapes (e.g., Kilburg, Nathan, & Thoreson, 1986; Mahoney, 1997; Sussman, 1995; Thoreson, Bud, & Krauskopf, 1986). Flight from reality in the arms of unhealthy diversions is a form of the neurotic paradox: avoidance brings short-term relief but long-term misery. False cures do more than just make you feel good; they also provide a temporary escape from feeling badly about yourself (Baumeister, 1992).

Studies on psychotherapists' personal problems yield the following top 10: irritability, emotional exhaustion, insufficient or unsatisfactory sleep, loneliness, isolation, depression, anxiety, relationship conflicts, concerns about caseloads, and self-doubt about therapeutic effectiveness (Mahoney, 1997). Sound familiar? Given these difficulties, it is not surprising that any of us would be vulnerable to unhealthy escapes.

Of the infinite number of ways we can mistreat our distress, three seem to capture an inordinate number of mental health professionals. With no claim to exhaustiveness, let us briefly review substance abuse, isolation, and sexual acting out. In each case, please perform an honest appraisal of your own self-care and identify whether the problem applies to you. Our aim in this section is to help you identify and begin altering unhealthy escapes that might hurt you and your patients.

Substance Abuse

Arguably the most prevalent self-destructive escape among psychotherapists is substance abuse (Guy, 1987). The incidence of alcohol and drug abuse among psychotherapists is alarmingly high, according to even the most conservative estimates (Kilburg et al., 1986; Thoreson et al., 1986;

Sussman, 1995). While substance abuse results from multiple causes, Thoreson and colleagues (1986) found that several practice factors relate to its development:

- Heightened personal insight and self-discovery, which can tempt some to experiment with psychoactive drugs.
- Feelings of grandiosity resulting from clinical practice, leading to denial or minimization of the symptoms of substance misuse and its associated risks.
- Lack of supervision from colleagues or supervisors, allowing the therapist to conceal the presence and impact of drugs from others.
- Little threat of job loss in independent practice, allowing for greater impairment before legal or professional sanctions are imposed.
- Work-related accomplishments that can conceal the deleterious effects that substance abuse has on the therapist's ability to conduct psychotherapy.

Risk factors for developing substance abuse are aggravated by psychotherapists' perceived barriers to care. Psychotherapists who think they may have a problem with alcohol, illicit drugs, and/or prescription drugs are often resistant to seek substance abuse evaluations, formal treatment, or 12-step programs. Perceived barriers to care include inflated fears of harming their professional reputations once the shameful secret is shared with others. As one psychotherapist argued, "What if one of my colleagues or patients saw me at an AA [Alcoholics Anonymous] meeting? I know so many people, it is bound to happen!"

Isolation

Psychotherapists are often physically and psychologically isolated—alone with our clients in a small soundproof room, separating ourselves from the outside world during the workday. No visitors, no phone calls, no interruptions during sessions. In between sessions, we remain physically isolated as we write notes or dictate reports in a quiet office. We have also fine-tuned the skill of psychic isolation—being emotionally subsumed in our clients—and are committed to protecting their secrets.

Even when we are not working, the long hours spent conducting assessments and therapy can breed further isolation outside of the office, as discussed in Chapter 3. How easy it is for this self-segregation to spill over into our personal lives (e.g., Farber, 1983b; Mahoney, 1997). Perhaps the most serious result of physical and psychic isolation is the therapist's increasing inability to overcome these restraints in her own private life. In other words, the very factors associated with the healer role that promote a sense of loneliness and separation in professional relations carry over into personal interactions as well. This is often due to the fact that the practicing psychotherapist finds it difficult to set aside the professional role outside of the office (Guy, 1987).

If we are not on guard against the tendency to isolate ourselves, we quickly begin avoiding contact with family and friends as a way of coping (Margison, 1987). As one psychotherapist described it:

> "After listening to patients and staff talk *to* me all day, when I leave the office, the last thing I want to do is listen to my family or friends. I understand they all have something they want to discuss with me, but by the time I get out of the office, it's like my brain has reached maximum storage capacity for verbal input, and I have no space for any one else to "download" onto me. The only way I can get some quiet time to decompress is to isolate when I get home."

While the lure of isolating to cope with feeling overwhelmed or overstimulated is certainly understandable, too little time with our family and friends places our well-being in harm's way.

Stop and ask yourself: Are you becoming less inclined to watch local or national broadcasts? Do you make an effort to listen to contemporary music? Watch new feature films? Read popular books? How isolated have you become?

Sexual Acting Out

Literature reviews point to a disturbingly high incidence of sexual acting out among therapists (Sussman, 1995). Coupled with the alarming percentage of psychotherapists, overwhelmingly male, having sexual relations with patients or students (e.g., Pope & Bouhoutsos, 1986; Pope, Sonne, & Holroyd, 1993), the research strongly suggests that sex is a powerful temptation for the distressed or impaired therapist. Sexual activity has all of the reinforcing effects created by recreational drugs: physical pleasure, exhilaration, tension release, relaxation, a temporary flight from reality, and ego enhancement. But, as indicated by a growing body of literature, sexual activity with clients is also a dangerous escape from emptiness, unresolved conflict, or a need for power.

Why are psychotherapists easy candidates for sexual acting out? For one, checking our professional hat at the door is often a difficult transition, thus requiring a certain degree of deliberation. Since we spend the majority of our professional time in the role of healer, it is not surprising when this role contaminates our romantic relationships. And reciprocally, romantic relationships can contaminate our therapeutic relationships. For another, many of us enter the profession out of an altruistic desire to eradicate mental health suffering, that of our patients and ourselves. Sometimes these desires can manifest themselves in sexual responses and rescue fantasies. Support for this phenomenon comes from the high percentage of therapists reporting fantasies about their patients—sexual and rescue-oriented in nature—at some point in their careers (Edelwich & Brodsky, 1991; Kottler, 1993).

Sexual feelings often arise in psychotherapy relationships, occasioned in the patient, the therapist, or simultaneously. Since this remains a taboo topic in training and supervision, therapists often miss the early warning signs that boundary violations with patients are looming or occurring. Many psychotherapists are simply not trained to effectively intervene before sexual acting out has taken place (Pope, Sonne, & Greene, 2006). Whatever the confluence of causes, it is ultimately the therapist's choice and responsibility, not the other person in the dyad. Simply stated, we must guard against acting on such feelings with our patients.

It behooves us all to complete a self-assessment of unhealthy escapes and to participate in supervision and treatment, as needed. In the spirit in which *Leaving It at the Office* was written, you can approach these tasks in an unabashedly human and accepting fashion. As a psychotherapist, if you are engaging in these or other destructive escapes, we implore you to search within yourself to discover what you are experiencing internally, what you are avoiding, what you need to address. Please seek the assistance of your peers, supervisors, and personal therapists. Once you have determined your unmet needs, then you can take measures that will eradicate the symptoms instead of masking them.

HEALTHY ESCAPES AT THE OFFICE

Adaptive escapes from the burdens of the office begin, paradoxically, at the office. Brief renewing escapes can be blended into your day, in between patients or between professional responsibilities. There are dozens of healthy paths to escaping the strains of our impossible profession; here, we offer a variety of self-care methods designed to assist therapists during the workday by engaging in good, clean escapism.

Vital Breaks

In the busyness of our day, it might seem counterproductive to slow down or to take a break. On the other hand, as we frequently remind our patients, it is no more a waste of time than stopping to put gas in our car when the tank is almost empty. It is necessary, it is beneficial. Taking breaks can create more time and energy. A growing body of research underscores the imperative of creating time for periodic escape in order for us to maintain psychological equilibrium (Carroll et al., 1999; Kottler, 1993; Ryan, 1999; Shoyer, 1999).

Most of us have made great strides in our career by overextending ourselves—holding 10 therapy sessions back-to-back, skipping lunches, and working 12-hour days. Most of us hear a little voice in the back of our heads saying, "Me? Take a break? What a joke! I don't have *time* to take a break!" Such beliefs may be driven by our overachieving heritage and the implicit assumption that putting the patient first means putting ourselves last. We routinely encounter colleagues who insist that they cannot possibly take a 2-hour lunch break with colleagues, go to the gym after work, or schedule a 2-week vacation. We collegially disagree.

Relaxation

In a job as absorbing and demanding as ours, we need periodic relaxation *during* the workday—not simply after the workday. Relaxation reciprocally inhibits (or counterconditions) anxiety and tension. Some form of anti-stress restoration is particularly indicated for therapists who have habituated themselves to hectic schedules, physiological arousal, and overactive minds.

Relaxation at the office demonstrably improves the energy, empathy, and attention of psychotherapists. In his *Principles of Psychology* (1910, p. 424) William James writes: "the faculty of voluntary bringing back of a wandering attention over and over again is the very root of judgement, character, and will. . . . An education which should improve this faculty would be *the* education *par excellence*" (italics in original).

Our master clinicians assuredly concur. One observes:

"I am involved in many types of meditation, including tai chi and yoga. Probably my favorite is tai chi, because it is very fluid and involves motion rather than just quiet sitting. The important factor when you do tai chi is to focus on your breath and to move in concert with your breath. As a clinician we are always focusing on others. We are supposed to be the mirror who shows them who they really are. Taking that stance all day leaves us little room to know who we are, how we feel, and what is important to us. Through focusing on my breath [during the workday], I become more aware of who I am and that I am a vital living being. [Meditation in the office] helps me to feel closer to humanity, and this helps me develop empathy in my practice."

Relaxation takes many forms. The most common among psychotherapists in the office are brief meditations, muscle relaxation, and deep breathing. But any activity that reduces our autonomic and mental activity—music, imagery, a few moments of pleasant reading—will certainly invoke a relaxation response. Make relaxation part of your work.

Humor

Laughter is a universal elixir: it helps us recover from physical maladies, mental distress, and emotional pain. In one study of psychotherapists (Kramen-Kahn & Hansen, 1998), maintaining a sense of humor was the most frequently endorsed career-sustaining behavior (82% endorsement). As Mark Twain, one of the world's most celebrated humorists, said in *The Mysterious Stranger* (1897):

> The human race, in its poverty, has unquestionably one really effective weapon: Laughter. Power, money, supplication and persuasion . . . these can lift a colossal humbug, they can lift poverty a little, century by century. . . . But only laughter can blow it to rags and atoms at a blast. Against the assault of laughter no evil can stand.

The utility of humor in therapy began with Freud, who wrote extensively on the subject (Barron, 1999). In the past 25 years or so, an increasing number of psychotherapists have been seeking both theoretical and empirical evidence to support incorporating humor into the psychotherapeutic transaction (Bloch, Browning, & McGrath, 1983; Goldstein, 1982; Heuser, 1980). Humor is typically used in stressful workplaces to counter anxiety, frustration, fear, and puzzlement. Common antecedents for practitioner use of humor are novel behaviors, bizarre thoughts, negative evaluations of self and role, and perceived threats to physical well-being (Warner, 1991). The growing body of empirical research supports the nation that humor in psychotherapy is decidedly beneficial (Cann, Holt, & Calhoun, 1999; Goldin & Bordin, 1999).

Humor in therapy profits both the therapist and the client. Beyond providing us with entertainment and allowing us to share the joy of laughter, humor also reduces tension, discharges energy, lifts affect from despair and suffering, provides intellectual stimulation, puts events in perspective, stimulates creative thinking, deals with the incongruous, the sublime, the awkward, and the nonsensical, broaches difficult subjects in less threatening ways, expresses exuberance and warmth, and creates a bond between those sharing a joke.

In addition to the benefits of using humor during the therapeutic process itself, a sense of humor outside of therapy sessions can assist the therapist in coping with painful sessions and frustrating patients (Parrish & Quinn, 1999). A master clinician, who directs an agency, offers examples:

"Something that really helps is to find ways to build humor into your work. One thing that we did all began with the purchase of the book *The Little Brown Dictionary of Anecdotes*, which was edited by Clifton Fadiman. We rotate who runs staff meetings, and everybody takes their turn. When you run the staff meeting, you get to pick a couple of anecdotes to read. People can't wait for us to get to the anecdotes, moving through the business items quickly to get to them. [Another] thing all of our staff try to learn is to tell a few jokes and cut the edge of the thing, whether it be a staff or clinical issue. We've also taken highly stressful or confusing events and changed them into skits. We sometimes play one out of something that at the time was not real funny but in retrospect is."

Sometimes we laugh with our clients, sometimes we laugh privately afterward, and sometimes we share the laughter with our colleagues. A master clinician offered this illustration:

"I am blind and use a seeing-eye dog. I was counseling a shy young guy, probably about 18 years old. He was talking about how hard it was for him to make contact with people. We were doing okay, but you could tell he was really struggling to talk. Then he got an itch in his private parts, which all of us do from time to time. He assessed the situation and figured that, since I was blind, I would not know what he was doing, and he took care of his itch. He sat there and scratched his itch. My ears really localize sound, so I knew exactly what he was doing. But I knew that, if I even smiled, he would be out of there because he was so shy. I was biting my lips to keep a straight face. He finishes the session, and I go running down the hall to tell one of my colleagues."

A therapist's sense of humor is a reflection of her joyfulness, passion, creativity, and playfulness. It allows us to cope more sanely with such intensely serious subjects. A good laugh may be the best tool available to help us let go and put our current situation into perspective. And, as one of our master clinicians put it, "If you are not having fun or if you're not able to laugh at yourself, you're in trouble."

Get-Togethers

Healthy escapes at the office are not limited to solo pursuits. Inviting your colleagues, staff members, friends, or family members to join you serves several functions. First, it allows you to socialize, to share stories and life events, to laugh, or to just hang out. Your workplace becomes associated not only with the grueling work but also with fun and socialization. Second, group activities allow many to reap the rewards of taking time off for frolicking. Third, due to the structured nature of our work, getaways help break up the routine of our day. They are vital breaks in the day, as discussed earlier in the chapter.

Spontaneous escapes are sometimes the most rewarding. Consider the following from one of our master therapists:

> "We will take the staff out to fun events. We'll pick some place to go out and take an excursion. For example, one afternoon, we had a succession of difficult client situations in which you know you just can't win. Also we had a stretch where everybody had very busy schedules and a number of staff members had things go wrong in their families and personal lives. They were coming to work a little bit down to start with, and then all this stuff was happening, and everybody was feeling overwhelmed. There was a sense that no one was on top of their game. We basically just said let's get the hell out of here. Sometimes the best time to shut down is when you're busiest. We went to get some tea. It was just a very nice break."

Such retreats from the office can also be planned in advance, as another testimonial attests:

> "We make it a point to try to celebrate accomplishments or people's time here. While that doesn't sound like a big deal, what I have found over many years is that in mental health services, if there is any area people are deficient in, it's how to celebrate and how to do positive things. The other day we took the whole staff to a new art exhibit. In the winter we have had fun in the sun parties. The staff will set up a fake beach and a heat lamp. Then we'll play Hawaiian music, and people will come in costumes like wetsuits and skin-diving outfits. It's meant to get rid of winter at its worst part."

Vital breaks, relaxation, humor, and get-togethers are healthy escapes at the office that allow us to decompress. Along with nurturing relationships (Chapter 5) and diverse professional activities (Chapter 12), such self-care at the office is precisely what the psychotherapist ordered after a long day, during a hectic week, or amid a busy season.

HEALTHY ESCAPES AWAY FROM THE OFFICE

Research has identified the broad strategy of counterconditioning—what we characterize as healthy escapes—as a reliable predictor of effective self-care among mental health practitioners. Whether you directly ask clini-

cians to tell you what maintains their well functioning or indirectly corre-
late their in-session behavior with their subsequent mood, healthy escapes
are always popular. Classic modes of escape include humor, vacations,
relaxation, self-assertion, cognitive restructuring, exercise, and diversion—
all action-oriented activities incompatible with occupational anxiety. Having already considered exercise in Chapter 4 ("Minding the Body"), assertion in Chapter 6 ("Setting Boundaries"), and cognitive restructuring in
Chapter 7 ("Restructuring Cognitions"), here we focus on examples and
advice related to other escapes outside of the office. In this chapter, we
enjoin you, quite literally, to leave it at the office.

Any strenuous or absorbing activity, in principle, can serve as an
effective means of escape (Baumeister, 1992). Literally to "let go" of the
burden of one's professional self, to escape the tyranny of work-related
burdens, to be liberated from the fetters of selfhood. In other words, to
escape *from* the burdens of the impossible profession and to escape *to*
absorbing errands, as Henry James advised at the chapter's opening.

The research supports the obvious: "Any group of people whose
selves are linked to high standards or expectations, or who are constantly
threatened with loss of face, will tend to be exposed to greater ego stress
and will therefore have a greater need of periodic escapes" (Baumeister,
1992, p. 34). Sound familiar?

Here are a dozen quick examples of healthy escapes away from the
office from our workshop participants and our therapist colleagues:

- Crocheting for charity. It's concrete. It's appreciated. It's with a
  group of people who have nothing to do with psychology.
- Taking up a new hobby, just for the fun of it and just for me. I'm
  learning to build furniture. Got myself a router. Made sawdust.
  Fun!
- Went to the [Florida] Keys in search of the mighty tarpon. Landed
  one and jumped three others. These behemoths are a hoot on a fly
  rod. My fishing buddy and I fished hard, drank hard, and behaved
  in politically incorrect and deeply immature ways. It was a great
  time.
- One of my favorite out-of-town escapes is to go kayaking. When you
  are on the water or sitting on an island that can only be accessed by
  boat, your voicemail and difficult therapy cases feel very far away. I
  always feel refreshed and ready to return to the complexity of work
  after such an adventure.
- Five pages of Proust every morning.
- A healthy escape from the office is to spend time reading. I read a
  mixture of professional material and books purely for enjoyment
  and entertainment. To this end I have joined a book club that keeps
  me in the habit of reading.

- Doing nothing! Just relaxing by myself without demands, anxieties, or other people.
- I am taking weekly violin lessons. I had never played a string instrument, but I love the violin. When I play *Twinkle, Twinkle, Little Star* or *My Pony* and other elementary tunes, I feel so good inside. This is a gentle self-care activity, quite different from the hard exercise I usually engage in to reduce my stress.
- My favorite form of healthy escape is becoming involved in my child's activities, such as school recitals, academic competitions, athletic games, and good old-fashioned horseplay. I also volunteer at the school when my schedule allows, and I join [my son] there for lunch a few times a year. Spending time with my son is the quickest route of diversion for me, as I am instantly transformed from therapist to mommy.
- Caring for a family of special-needs cats and dogs who live in our home.
- For expression, I write with a pen and paper each morning, and I paint on canvas. When I yearn for connection to my ancestors, I cook the recipes of my mother, of my grandmother, and of her mother.

Such examples can serve as portals to sensitivity and depth—or can confine us to meaningless particulars if pursued to obsessional lengths (Sacks, 1985). In the following pages, we endeavor to synthesize the idiographic with the nomothetic, the particulars and the general, in developing healthy escapes outside of the office.

Day(s) Off

We all require a Shabbat—a regularly scheduled day of rest and respite from the week's demands. This is a day designed for peace and spirituality, a separate time to focus on family, friends, relaxation, and spirituality. It need not be a Saturday or Sunday, but it needs to be a genuine day off.

One of our master clinicians offers this remedy:

"Despite, or perhaps because of, our hectic schedules, my family and I enjoy taking quick minivacations on the weekends. As luck would have it, these getaways are usually located on the beach—one of my favorite places to escape from the stressors of life. Sometimes we have a destination in mind, but at other times we just throw a few things in a bag, load up the car, and drive south. This is always an adventure!"

Many psychotherapists are on call 7 days a week. We strongly advise them to reconsider this policy, to give themselves a Shabbat. If you are available 24/7 to your patients, you are never truly available to yourself and your significant others.

Vacations

American workers generally get a measly 2 weeks of vacation per year, among the lowest of industrialized nations. Even so, many Americans do not use all of their vacation time or days. To complicate matters further, we are sometimes actively discouraged or prohibited from taking the entire 2 weeks at the same time. Then we're frequently asked to be accessible during the vacation!

Follow Freud's example: take a month of vacation per year, away from the office, and largely out of contact. Be away—physically, mentally, emotionally. As one colleague confessed, "It took me a day or two to remember how to play!" Many of us do not even begin to relax on vacation until 3 days into it and then begin to worry about our awaiting workload 2 days before the end of vacation. The restorative function of vacations may take a full 2 weeks.

For those who immediately protest "But I can't afford it!" we offer the wise words of distinguished psychologist Arnold Lazarus. He (2000, p. 93) pointedly argues that "avarice and greed are responsible for most of the stressors that beset many professionals." He—and we—know that far too many psychotherapists are greedy, working more than 60 hours a week, mainly for the money. Lazarus, by contrast, deliberately allows time for leisure and vacations. "A basic goal in my life has never been to make money—only to earn a decent living. My bank account may have suffered, but my psyche has been enriched."

If longer vacations are not feasible, we highly recommend taking minivacations throughout the year. Imagine all the places that you can escape to within just a few hours! Take advantage of your location and the many places that remain unexplored.

When we get away from our offices, our patients, and our colleagues, we regain a perspective on what is truly important in our lives. And, as Kottler (1993) points out, "Eventually there comes a time when we grow tired of living out of a suitcase and feel ready, if not eager, to return to that which we call work."

Leisurely Diversions

Two of the most frequent ways in which psychotherapists attempt to prevent distress are to take periodic vacations and to participate in non-work-related activities (Sherman & Thelen, 1998). About 9 in 10 of us do so.

In one of our studies (Hoeksma et al., 1993), as should surprise no one, psychotherapists' satisfaction with their leisure activities was significantly correlated with decreased burnout. In fact, about 10% of burnout symptoms could be accounted for by respondents' paucity of leisure activities.

The range of therapists' nonvocational leisure activities is impressive (Burton, 1969, 1972). Whether it is reading, creative outlets, hobbies, or travel, the vast majority of psychotherapists enjoy getting away from it all, both figuratively and literally.

In our self-care research and workshops, we have been impressed with the ubiquity of psychotherapists gravitating to simple and concrete leisure activities. "I really enjoy cutting the lawn," "Working in my wood shop," or "I love puttering in the garden" are frequent refrains. Psychotherapy is a sedentary, diffuse activity with ambiguous indicators of delayed outcomes. The ideal counterweight is concrete physical activity with clearly visible and obvious outcomes. Many of us have taken to heart *Chop Wood, Carry Water* (Field, 1984)—a famous Buddhist book. The chores get us out of our heads, thus balancing and centering us.

Novelty also figures prominently into leisure activities. A master clinician offers this advice, pointing out that she prefers:

> " . . . novel activities, like go on a mystery night on a cruise ship, have a theme party at the house, travel to unusual places, go out with the most interesting people I can find who are not in psychology (so I don't hear psychology talk). I might do some unconventional things where I don't have to act professionally. Because of the small town I live in, people always know who you are. Spending time away from where I practice so I don't always have to be at my most professional always helps."

Take music, for a prominent example. Music is one of the most effective escapes known to humankind. A number of clinical and experimental studies show that music has many therapeutic benefits (Sloboda, 1999), such as greater positivity (e.g., more happy), greater arousal (e.g., more alert), and greater present-mindedness (e.g., less bored). Better still, music can also be combined with many other healthy escapes—exercise, relaxation, play, and solitude.

Two of our master therapists tell us:

> "My favorite way of escaping is through listening to music. The music I listen to can facilitate the release of most emotions—from sadness, remorse, frustration, and anger to happiness, joy, optimism, and acceptance. When I leave a day of conducting therapy, I typically experience some combination of these feelings. I listen to music and sing in my car on the way home, and it helps me work through these feelings before I get home. I find it very easy to escape into music."

"I love music. It is one of the easiest ways for me to immerse and cleanse my mind throughout the day. I listen to it most of the time that I am alone, whether I am writing or running or cooking dinner. I might also jump up and do a little dance if I am alone. It gives me a boost in energy and lifts my mood like nothing else. It is also a hobby of mine. As a result, I have quite an extensive collection of music to choose from to fit my current mood and activities."

Thoughtfully chosen music can indeed be restful, relaxing, and renewing. Find which kind of music works for you for specific occasions. Need more energy or motivation? Try playing music with a fast beat, dramatic pieces, or something from your youth. Want to lift your mood? Listen to songs or tunes that trigger memories of your most positive experiences or other carefree eras in your life. Need to wind down? Try putting on something with a slower melody. Need something conducive to being totally present in the moment? Try Eckhart Tolle's *Gateways to Now* or other CDs that focus our minds and help us meditate.

Restorative Solitude

Lest our examples appear to focus on social activities, let us be clear about the balance between socialization and alone time. After taxing days filled with demanding interpersonal interactions with patients, students, and administrators, many of us crave solitude.

When was the last time you were away by yourself—truly alone—for 24 hours? Forty-eight hours? Ever? We are in almost constant contact with others—and need to be for emotional and practical reasons. Yet, time spent alone is an essential biological and developmental need for all of us to maintain our mental health (Buchholz, 1997; Hoff & Buchholz, 1996). In fact, some argue that a lack (not an abundance) of solitude leads to maladaptive behavior.

Of course, the optimal balance between interpersonal contact and restorative solitude is an individual matter, affected by our personality style, work demands, and so on. One of us prefers little socialization after lengthy clinical days; the other prefers nondemanding fun after lengthy clinical days. Psychotherapists working in a hospital or community setting where face-to-face contact hours are greater, and opportunities for breaks are fewer, seem to favor more solitude away from the office.

We are avid practitioners of double-dipping on healthy escapes. We exercise with friends, we vacation with family, and we engage in a multitude of "twofers" escapes. In this respect, one added benefit of solitude is that it can be combined with other forms of healthy escapism—exercise, hobbies, relaxation, meditation, and traveling, to name a few.

Personal Retreats

Hours of restorative solitude can be extended into personal retreats. Retreats promise geographic, emotional, and interpersonal solace. One of our colleagues took a ferry from southern Rhode Island to Block Island in the morning, spent the night in a local hotel, and devoted the day and a half to himself, before returning to a delicious lobster dinner seaside with his family. It was an opportunity for dedicated reflection, discernment, and renewal.

During retreats, some colleagues prefer directed exercises, such as the spiritual exercises of St. Ignatius, while others prefer stream-of-consciousness journaling and meditation. Some prefer established retreat centers with fellow travelers on similar journeys, while still others prefer the anonymity and separateness of a Holiday Inn 80 miles from their home. The external attributes of the getaway are not nearly as important as the internal process: dedicated reflection and renewal as a person and, thus, as a psychotherapist.

"Human kind cannot bear very much reality," as T. S. Eliot (1992, p. 118) reminds us. A psychotherapist relates:

> I go into the desert to get lost. And lately, I can't get lost often enough. I long for the moment when I can get behind the wheel of my four-wheel drive and aim the tires for a spot out there where my body runs on automatic pilot, and the dust of the desert clears my brain of city dust and haze, of tobacco and caffeine, and all the things that therapists absorb from their environment. . . . Here [in the desert], I don't spend time, I have time; for the days in the desert are longer, the nights are real nights when I can lie back and count stars the way an insomniac counts sheep. (Fox, 1998, p. 104)

On such retreats or vacations, we encourage you to leave your professional role at home by avoiding requests to talk shop or proffer advice. In fact, when one of us vacations and travels, he fudges and characterizes himself as a "consultant" or a "teacher" to avoid the ubiquitous requests for psychological information or assistance. Politely responding with "I don't practice outside of the office" rarely suffices; a bit of dissembling is required to stop the assaults on our personal time. It's a small white lie of omission but a small moral price to pay for self-care and renewal.

We are enthusiastic about personal retreats, but ambivalent about mandatory all-office retreats in which all clinicians from the same agency or clinic take the day or weekend. First, such retreats tend to be mandatory and thus another imposition of control. Second, the retreat agenda is typically the administration's or management's, not clinicians'. Third, it intrudes into personal time. Of course, these concerns can be rectified if practitioners run the retreat, collaborate on the agenda and goals, and are paid for work time. In general, we advocate personal retreats, not office retreats, or organized retreats for renewal of health care professionals, which we see advertised and offered all around the country.

Personal retreats can be lengthened into clinical sabbaticals (Freudenberger & Robbins, 1979), taking a month, or a couple of months, away from clinical responsibilities. The disadvantages are obvious: interruption of patient care, loss of income, disruption of referrals, and so on. Nonetheless, we are among those who favor clinical sabbaticals every 3–5 years.

Play

One of our favorite questions in self-care workshops is "How do you play?" How do you step away from a busy life, have fun, and find renewal?

The emerging answers come in two varieties. The first answer, from about three-quarters of psychotherapists, is that they play in a multitude of ways impossible to catalogue. They play as hard as they work at every imaginable activity. They paint, write, sing, dance, fish, watch movies, exercise, and perform as clowns at birthday parties (we kid you not). Many point to their hobbies as self-nourishing, playful escapes from work and into their passions. We distinctly recall one workshop participant who proclaimed that his 2–3 hours a week at his potter's wheel was his "salvation." These nonrational and creative pursuits counterbalance the typically serious and rational nature of conducting psychotherapy. Such pursuits free the therapist from the burdensome compulsion of attempting to understand patients and solve problems (Boylin & Briggie, 1987).

The second answer to "How do you play?"—from the remaining one-quarter of psychotherapists—is that "I don't." A typical response is "Well, I don't really play. I used to, but then work, kids, mortgages, and life took my time and energy. It's tough enough just working."

Our immediate response is profoundly empathic. Life in general, and the practice of psychotherapy in particular, can certainly rob us of the inclination to play. We have all been confronted with these strains and can all feel the burden. At the same time, we cannot help but feel a sadness that once vital people are stagnant, that they and their loved ones are robbed of joyful vitality. Our next response is to gently inquire how we might get that playful feeling and commitment back into their lives.

What ways did you used to play? What sports are fun and remind you of the carefree days of your youth? Some ideas that come to mind: amusement rides, water slides, water-gun fights, hide-and-seek, blowing bubbles, catching fireflies, playing horseshoes, volleyball, basketball, or baseball. Building structures out of clay, sand, or dirt. Running through the pouring rain—and jumping in the mud puddles! Playing board games—especially the ones that include acting, drawing, or building. Playing a musical instrument. Dancing around the living room. Singing in the car. The possibilities are limitless.

For the three-quarters or so of you, please keep playing and playing hard! Feel rejuvenated without the professional burdens. For the other one-quarter, please learn to turn off the professional role so that you can be spontaneous, joyful, even immature at times. Relearn the power of play.

Reading and Writing

Most psychotherapists have several books in them: books about their clinical experiences, interesting patients, life lessons, and messages of renewal, as well as fictional works that might capitalize on their keen observational skills, writing ability, and creative imagination. We love writing and reading for fun.

Some of us record our dreams, others journal as self-care, some write fiction, and some carry notebooks and jot down phrases and quotes (how did you think all of these found their way into this book?!). The writing genre is probably not as important as the act of creative expression itself. Find a writing outlet for self-care.

Few pleasures rival curling up in a comfy chair with a good book after a draining workday. Lost in fiction or reading biographies, psychotherapists revel in the sheer pleasure of ideas, narratives, fantasy, and adventure. Some of us prefer trashy, I-don't-have-to-think novels and others the intellectual challenge of mystery. In all cases, reading gives us pleasure and respite.

Humor

Humor is used not only to facilitate the therapeutic process but also to nurture the individual clinician. Humor is a perfect antidote for the stresses of the occupation, the crippling disorders of some of our patients, and our occasional pomposity. Serious humor researchers find that it is powerful medicine that offers a panoply of health benefits. Laughter increases oxygen flow, elevates mood, encourages relaxation, provides an analgesic effect, and likely has a detectable beneficial effect on immune functioning (Martin, 2001). A sense of humor has been shown, in rigorous prospective analyses (e.g., Nezu, Nezu, & Blissett, 1988), to serve as a stress buffer. It is an effective, mature coping mechanism that prevents distress.

Consider the following two pieces of levity, shared repeatedly in private conversations or faxed repeatedly from one clinician to another. A single-frame cartoon shows the stereotypical male psychotherapist, with a couch in the background, slapping the hapless patient across the face and ordering him to "Snap out of it!" The caption reads "Single-Session Therapy."

The second item is a joke: A wealthy and aggressive managed-care executive meets with his demise and finds himself standing in front of St. Peter at the pearly gates. The executive is understandably consumed with anxiety and apologizes profusely. St. Peter looks benignly upon the man and renders the verdict "You may enter heaven . . . " The managed-care executive, relieved and overjoyed, runs through the pearly gates into his heavenly reward. But then St. Peter finishes, "but just for 3 days."

In these two pieces of levity, we find classic expressions of aggression sublimated into mature humor. In the case of the cartoon, feeling pressured by the finances of short-term treatment, psychotherapists chuckle appreciatively at the potential horror and downright violence they envision for the ultimate in single-session psychotherapy. In the case of the joke, feeling displaced as arbitrators of patient health care and contemptuous of the unconscionable salaries of managed-care executives, psychotherapists revel in the "just desserts" of the executive's receiving the same (limited) treatment afforded to many of our valued clients.

Of course, humor can be misused, as in attempts to dominate, evade, or laugh *at* instead of *with* others. It must be sensitively and properly applied. And when it is, humor is as restorative as sleep, in which we "burst into" health-giving benefits.

Meditation

Earlier in this chapter we discussed brief relaxation and meditative escapes at the office, but here we underscore the point that many mental health practitioners have adopted meditation as a lifestyle outside of the office.

Meditation is a simple process, if one can set aside the need for accomplishment and goals. Meditative escapes bring relief by rejecting ordinary thoughts and adopting a serene observational stance. The various meditative techniques disrupt the mind's tendency to jabber on about everything that happens and to analyze it ad infinitum. Meditation involves letting ordinary thoughts come and go without judgment, interference, or disruption. By abandoning egotism and adopting a pervasive attitude of modesty, practitioners can avoid the burden of having to keep an overgrown, overvalued self up to inflated standards (Baumeister, 1992). The broader philosophical-cognitive shift that life is suffering—the first of Buddha's Four Noble Truths—can help us abort the extended "pity parties" we throw for ourselves. Meditation clears the mind, refreshes the spirit, and centers us through close connection with the physical world.

One of our master clinicians describes his meditative escape this way:

"About 6 months ago, I realized that my ambitious and driven behavior was taking a toll on me—physically, emotionally, and spiritually. I knew that I had to find some way to slow myself down. I wanted to find something that I could do just for myself—not for my family, not for my clients, and not for my vitae. So I began meditating. Each day, I make the time to meditate. Periods of sitting motionless and intensely focusing my mind calm my thinking, lift my mood, and soothe my soul."

AND A COLLEGIAL WARNING

Our research studies have identified not only what predicts effective self-care but also what predicts ineffective self-care—the "to do" as well as the "not to do." This chapter has been occupied almost exclusively with the former, so before we close we should attend to the latter.

Two strategies are reliably associated with self-care *in*effectiveness among psychotherapists (Norcross & Aboyoun, 1994) and among the population at large (Penley, Tomoka, & Wiebe, 2002): *wishful thinking* and *self-blame*. By focusing on not being able to change and relying on wishing rather than acting, the frequent use of wishful thinking probably accentuates distress and reduces problem solving. In a similar way, the negative preoccupation of self-blame may distress the therapist further and paralyze adaptive recourses. The moral is simple: avoid wishful thinking and self-blame.

In our experience, many psychotherapists suffering a paucity of healthy escapes may wind up engaging in wishful thinking and self-blame after listening to their colleagues in self-care workshops or reading this chapter. "My colleagues got their self-care acts together. What's wrong with me? I'm not nearly as creative or resourceful as my peers. I wish I could do those things too!" And, as workshop leaders, we are humbled and more than a little envious of the superstars of healthy escapes that we encounter.

When these and related thoughts happen to you, we would offer four collegial directions. First, please do not compare yourself to the glowing exemplar of self-care highlighted in a workshop or this chapter, but to the typical practitioner struggling to remain sane and solvent in a busy life. Second, remind yourself that healthy escapes are merely one strategy of self-care, and some of our colleagues who excel at leisurely diversions do little else for self-care. There is no single self-care strategy so outstandingly effective that its possession alone ensures health (as noted in Chapter 1). Having a particular hobby or leisure pursuit is less important than engaging in a variety of self-care strategies. Third, transform the wishful thinking into action—perhaps you are, in fact, in need of more escapes away from the office. Mobilize the self-blame in order to take constructive action. Fourth and finally, if chronically plagued by self-blame and wishful thinking, then please consider peer consultation (Chapter 5) and personal therapy (Chapter 10). This may well represent an enduring personality pattern, as opposed to a transient reaction.

IN CLOSING

How, exactly, do psychotherapists manage to take their minds off their professional identities and leave their distress at the office? The self cannot simply be turned off like a lamp (Baumeister, 1992). Creating healthy escapes requires a skillful attitude, an abiding commitment, and absorbing errands.

Healthy escapes must be defined and discovered individually; what one clinician classifies as self-care may be a stressor for another (Williams-Nickelson, 2006). For example, sports participation may be relaxing for some, but the competition is stressful for others. Some of us appreciate at least an hour of solitude each day, while others pursue interpersonal contact with nonclients. Or taking a family vacation may be relaxing for most, but not if you are the person responsible for coordinating every one else and then stuck with the extra work when you return. Determine what escape keeps you in touch with yourself.

Finding balance among love, work, and play is indispensable and yet probably overprescribed in the self-care literature. The advice is fine and well intentioned but results in little permanent change unless combined with some candid assessment of what purposes and meanings overwork has for you (Grosch & Olsen, 1994). If you exchange a few hours of compulsive overwork for a few hours of competitive exercising or compulsive hobbies, little has been accomplished. So, as we conclude the chapter, bear in mind that the advice must be combined with your own dynamics and vulnerabilities.

In this chapter, we offered a variety of healthy escapes to renew and energize you. To be sure, there are hundreds of other means not mentioned that you may find helpful in nurturing yourself. Our abiding hope is that this sampling will lead you to seek out or continue those escapes that work best for you.

But the greatest challenge in healthy escapism is not learning what works for you. The greatest challenge is building the practice into your daily life with regularity—both in and away from the office. As Henry James correctly observed at the beginning of this chapter, "The point is not only to get out—you've got to stay out; and to stay out you must have some absorbing errand."

SELF-CARE CHECKLIST

✓ Undertake a candid assessment of what purposes and significance overwork has for you. What really prevents you from engaging in healthy escapes?

✓ Perform an honest appraisal of *unhealthy* escapes (e.g., substance abuse, isolation, sexual acting out) and determine whether the problem applies to you.

✓ Make relaxation part of your workday; it improves your energy, empathy, and attention.

✓ Take vital breaks between patients and between clinical responsibilities.

✓ Maintain your sense of humor; it is a career-sustaining behavior.

✓ Join your colleagues and staff for get-togethers in the office and spontaneous escapes from it.

✓ Include phone calls, lunches, and breaks in your workday several times each week to provide contact with friends and family.

✓ Practice balance: over 80% of therapists routinely engage in reading or a hobby, take pleasure trips or vacations, and attend artistic events and movies as part of their self-care patterns (Mahoney, 1997).

✓ Schedule a weekly Shabbat—a regular day of rest and respite from the week's demands.

✓ Monitor your vacation time. Is it less than you as a psychotherapist would recommend to patients in similarly stressful occupations?

✓ Follow Freud's example: every year take several weeks away from the office, and stay largely out of contact.

✓ Create adventure and other diversions away from the office. Is play a steady staple of your emotional diet?

✓ "Chop wood, carry water": participate in concrete physical activities with a clearly visible and obvious outcome to counterbalance your psychotherapeutic work.

✓ Balance your socialization and alone time; determine how much restorative solitude you require.

✓ Take personal retreats that enable you to distance yourself geographically, emotionally, and interpersonally.

✓ Lengthen retreats into periodic clinical sabbaticals devoid of psychotherapy responsibilities.

✓ Reject ordinary thinking and adopt a more observational stance: Meditate.

✓ Try new and exciting activities for the first time: river rafting, camping, snorkeling, deep sea fishing, and the like.

✓ Avoid wishful thinking and self-blame in contemplating self-care; instead, pursue action-oriented strategies.

✓ Make a contract with yourself to integrate healthy escapes into your routine. Monitor and chart your progress.

✓ Ask yourself once a year (perhaps on your birthday), "How do I play?"

RECOMMENDED READING

Baumeister, R. F. (1992). *Escaping the self: Alcoholism, spirituality, masochism, and other flights from the burden of selfhood.* New York: Basic Books.

Fields, R. (1984). *Chop wood, carry water.* New York: Penguin.

Pope, K. S., Sonne, J. L., & Greene, B. (2006). *What therapists don't talk about and why: Understanding taboos that hurt us and our clients.* Washington, DC: American Psychological Association.

CHAPTER 9

Creating a
Flourishing Environment

Most recommendations to promote psychotherapist self-care and to prevent burnout fall into the category of changing the person (Maslach & Goldberg, 1998). This is essential and comprises much of the content of this book; however, it is incomplete. An exclusive focus on changing the person is too individualistic; it may erroneously blame the clinician; and it ignores the organizational and managerial factors that may cause the problem in the first place (Leiter & Maslach, 2005; Murphy & Pardeck, 1986).

In our research on self-care methods (e.g., Brady, Norcross, & Guy, 1995), psychotherapists rate "making organizational changes at the practice" their least frequently used method. It came in dead last among 27 self-care activities. Psychotherapists are far more comfortable and skilled in changing themselves than in changing the environment.

It is as though we are committing in our self-care the same fundamental attribution error we occasionally commit in our professional work. In arriving at causal attributions, we have a tendency to overestimate patient's dispositions and to underestimate the power of their situations. In other words, we are prone to weigh internal determinants too heavily and external determinants too lightly. We are thus likely to explain patients' behavior as resulting predominantly from their personality, while we often minimize (or even ignore) the importance of the particular environments in which they find themselves.

Let's correct the fundamental attribution error: harness the subtle but pervasive power of the environment to replenish yourself. Make the environment work for you, not against you.

We need to comprehensively address the person of the psychotherapist, the work environment, and their interaction. The workplace, the systems, the physical environment, the administration, and the sociocultural context—all are involved in the genesis and maintenance of self-care and the lack thereof. This is particularly true for mental health professionals working for clinics, agencies, hospitals, and other settings outside of private practices. Nonfunctional organizational factors contribute mightily to therapist distress and discourage responsible self-care.

In this chapter, we traverse the infrequently used but powerfully effective strategy of environmental control. Humans, unlike the nonhuman species on the planet, have enormous capacity to remake their environment. In the words of B. F. Skinner, "One can picture a good life by analyzing one's feelings, but one can only achieve it by arranging environmental contingencies." Make your working environment work in the cause of your self-care.

Again, the number of specific techniques for implementing the strategy is endless. For some, a flourishing environment might be aesthetics in your office decor; for others, replenishment in your refrigerator, nourishment from an administrator, or simply a humane caseload. This chapter is designed to assist you in refining or creating a flourishing environment.

PHYSICAL ENVIRONMENT

Let's begin with the tangible: the physical environment in which you work. What does it feel and look like? Attractive, soothing, and professional? Or, as is tragically the case in many public sectors, bland, irritating, and institutional?

Take an environmental audit of your work space. Consider the comfort and appeal of:

Wall paint	Lighting	Flooring
Ceiling	Ventilation	Windows
Smell or scent	Furniture	Artwork
Reading material	Waiting area	Music
Privacy	Safety	Neighborhood

Take Freud's workspace, for example. Although Freud was commonly regarded as a workaholic, his patients found that he possessed a special gift for creating a happy balance in everything he undertook, including the appearance of his home at Berggasse 19 (in Vienna). The Wolf-Man, one of Freud's more (in)famous analysands (in Gardiner, 1971, p. 137), writes:

> I can remember, as though I saw them today, his two adjoining studies, with the door open between them and with their windows opening on a little courtyard. There was always a feeling of sacred peace and quiet here. The rooms themselves must have been a surprise to any patient, for they in no way reminded one of a doctor's office but rather of an archeologist's study. Here were all kinds of statuettes and other unusual objects, which even the layman recognized as archeological finds from ancient Egypt. Here and there on the walls were stone plaques representing various scenes of long-vanished epochs. A few potted plants added life to the rooms, and the warm carpet and curtains gave them a homelike note. Everything here contributed to one's feeling of leaving the haste of modern life behind, of being sheltered away from one's daily cares.

You don't need to be a Freudian to learn from Freud: create a welcoming environment for patients and a flourishing environment for yourself. Soft colors, low lighting, cozy chairs, a lit candle, pleasant artwork, a fish tank, and soothing music go a long way in conveying comfort and privacy. One of our colleagues purchases a bunch of fresh flowers each week for his office. Physical improvements need not be expensive, just expansive.

SENSORY AWARENESS

Independent of the physical surroundings, we can cultivate our sensory awareness. Sensory diversion can help temporarily mollify nearly all forms of painful affect and replenish our overtaxed senses. Behold your surroundings using vision, hearing, touch, gustation, and olfaction. People pay good money to stay at beautiful vacation resorts; to hear mellifluous music, to acquire luxurious fabrics, to eat gourmet food, and to wear pleasant scents. Build these into your work environment.

As we try to increase our sensory awareness, look to children—the sensory masters. Children focus outward, not inward. On our way to adulthood and genuineness we have diminished the capacity to appreciate our surroundings. At times, our introspective nature can cause us to become so serious that we are oblivious to everything around us. Maybe we cannot fully recover the pristine senses of childhood; maybe, after exposing ourselves to the environment for so long, our neurons cannot "unlearn" what we have absorbed. However, we can teach ourselves to appreciate what used to come naturally: to observe and luxuriate in our environment.

A concrete (and inexpensive) method is to establish in the office a Refreshment Center. This center consists of mouthwash, cologne/perfume, brush, comb, washcloth, and so on to physically refresh us between appointments. If you have more than a drawer or file cabinet to spare, then also add water and fresh snacks to sustain you during the day (see also Chapter 4). Several of our colleagues fondly call this the Me Center—something clandestine just for them.

WORK SAFETY

In auditing the physical environment of your work, consider not simply comfort but the safety of the practice environment. Evidence is accumulating about the safety concerns of psychotherapists. In one of our nationwide surveys of psychotherapists, for example, 60% replied that they are often or sometimes concerned about unwanted calls to the office, 36% about unwanted calls to home, and 28% about verbal threats to personal safety (Guy et al., 1992). Concerns about physical attacks on one's self are, thankfully, appreciably lower—2% often and 20% sometimes, but still enough to be concerned.

The same study examined protective measures taken by psychotherapists (Guy et al., 1992). The most frequent were:

- Refusing to treat certain clients (50% said they had).
- Declining to disclose personal data to patients (41%).
- Prohibiting clients from appearing at their home (41%).
- Locating the office in a safe building (39%).
- Specifying intolerable patient behaviors (35%).

Other protective measures were to avoid working alone in the office, hiring a secretary, and installing an office alarm system. Although we covered this topic earlier (in Chapter 6, on setting boundaries), your physical safety is important enough to remind you to create a comfortable *and* safe practice environment.

BUSINESS SUPPORT

Psychotherapists don't enter the field because they are fascinated with its business aspects. We desire to be healers, not managers; helpers, not accountants.

One way to help therapists differentiate themselves from their practices is to ask them to imagine the practice as a distinct entity, something apart from themselves—another person, so to speak (Grodzki, 2003). Get distance and perspective on it.

When we can look at our practice in a dispassionate and distant manner, many times we conclude we are devoting inordinate time to dreaded, nonclinical responsibilities—the paperwork, the scheduling, the billing, the cleaning. In these instances, we recommend three paths or combinations thereof. First, hire office assistance for scheduling, billing, notes, taxes, authorizations, phone calls, the Internet, and other business aspects that you dislike or find nonproductive. Second, learn to streamline your office practices. Perform appointment scheduling as part of the session. Write uncomplicated notes. Minimize billing by insisting on payment each session or each month. Train staff members or the answering service to reduce interruptions and to do more of your paperwork. Third, if you are confused about the right path for you, hire a business coach or consult your accountant for cost-effective approaches to take. The goal is to maximize your time in what you enjoy and do well and to minimize what you deplore and others can do as well if not better than you.

Let me cite my own (JCN) personal history: Years ago, I learned that I was happier absorbing extra overhead expenses for my part-time practice in order to maintain a large, comfortable office and have an office manager handle all of the financial and billing matters. Yes, I net less private practice income as a result, but I enjoy my clinical work and therapy environment much more (Norcross, 2000).

Some self-care pundits urge practitioners to eliminate managed care entirely from their practices. It certainly reduces the business hassles of independent practice. We remain stridently ambivalent about this proposition. Personally, we do not participate in any managed care: one of us never accepted managed care, and the other purged it from his practice with pleasure. However, we are part-time practitioners with established practices who can afford to be selective. Such is simply not feasible for younger, full-time, and institutional practitioners. One-size-fits-all advice usually fits no one particularly well.

In all of these decisions, base your business decisions on love, not fear (Grodzki, 2003). Fear-based practice is loathsome, grim work, whereas love-based practice is grounded in love of the work and pride in your vocation. In fact, a therapist's sense of "feeling blessed" is most highly correlated with experiencing therapeutic work as healing involvement (Orlinsky & Rønnestad, 2005).

The foregoing chapters in *Leaving It at the Office* present multiple strategies for relieving the stress of personal depletion in conducting psychotherapy. But they do not deal directly with the management and business stressors most common to the independent practitioner, namely, time pressures, economic uncertainty, caseload uncertainty, and the business aspects of running a practice (Nash et al., 1984). These may best be handled by delegating them to administrative assistants, secretaries, office managers, billing services, or consultants. An irony is that we enter the healing professions in order to help people, only to find ourselves encumbered with endless paperwork. Create an environment where you spend your time and energies on what you like, and delegate the accompanying duties elsewhere.

BEHAVIORAL BOUNDARIES

Robert Sollod, a cherished colleague, was fond of exhorting colleagues to build "behavioral boundaries." He based this counsel on his studies of the shamanic traditions of separating healing from the rest of life through rituals. Shamans would perform an entry ritual in preparation for the healing—incense to purify, a little dance, spending a little time aside—and then later a closure ritual—cleansing, moving out of the space, being alone for a period of time.

Building behavioral boundaries entails temporarily separating yourself from the clinical world by means of routine and time. The routine between patients, or between your last patient and your personal time, might consist of going to the bathroom, washing hands, taking a nap, listening to music, or a lengthy commute. Give yourself time between patients. Ten or 15 minutes to make notes on the previous session, review notes of forthcoming session, return a call, stretch, breathe. It might lengthen your day and diminish your income, but as Irv Yalom (2002, p. 167) argues, "It is worth it." Extra time between patients may be poor time management, but it is definitely good stress management.

Insofar as you control your work environment, arrange it in your interest. Take control of your schedule. As we reviewed in Chapter 6, keep your caseload at a manageable level. Limit your practice to a specified number of high-risk and high-demand patients. Schedule the final patient of your day carefully. For one straight year, every Wednesday my (JCN) last patient in the evening was a woman who had lost her young child, her only child, to an automobile accident. She was suffering from unearthly grief and PTSD. Her pain left the office with me. Finally—remember, we do not profess to be experts in practicing self-care—we discovered that it was inadvisable to schedule her last in the day. Take more control over your schedule and build those behavioral boundaries.

INSTITUTIONAL PRACTICES

At this point in our workshops, participants are howling in their seats. "Hey, we don't have that kind of control at our clinic! We are assigned patients, and they are scheduled for us. What about us?" (Over the years, we have learned to anticipate these protests and state in advance that we will address these particular demands in a few moments.)

Practicing psychotherapy in institutional settings—clinics, hospitals, staff HMOs, centers, and various institutes—presents a host of encumbrances not afflicting independent practitioners. There are, simply put, fewer degrees of freedom.

In fact, the phenomenon of psychotherapist burnout was initially coined by Herb Freudenberger (1975) out of his work in an institutional setting. After a few years of unrealistic expectations, draining work schedules, mountains of paperwork, financial cutbacks, and working with severe mental illnesses, enthusiastic idealism slowly morphs into cynical detachment. The bright lightbulb has burned out.

In the worst of clinical institutions, practitioners are confronted with unresponsive management, lack of control, low staff–client ratios, insufficient rewards, inadequate funding, unrealistic demands for high productivity accompanied with little autonomy or flexibility, and ultimately a breakdown in the therapeutic community. No wonder that career dissatisfaction is highest and burnout most common among practitioners working in institutional settings (see also Chapter 2).

At the same time, the bulk of research indicates that it is neither the institutional setting itself nor the high demands alone that lead to psychotherapist stress. Highly demanding jobs can be made less stressful without lowering the amount of demands—so long as the level of constraints can be reduced and supports can be expanded. These results are consistent with the demands–supports–constraints model of occupational stress (Kramen-Kahn & Hansen, 1998). That is, clinical positions in institutional settings will continue to be demanding, but increasing the support and reducing the constraints make the positions rewarding and manageable.

Increasing practitioner support both inside and outside of the office has been covered in an entire chapter on nurturing relationships (Chapter 5). Support can take the form of clinical supervision, consultation, clinical teams, peer support, cuddle groups, and the like. In one study, the authors (Farber & Heifetz, 1982, p. 289) pointedly conclude that "most therapists found the role of support systems essential. All those who could utilized supervisory relationships to help them through difficult moments; of those who were not being supervised, 51.1% relied on informal support of colleagues."

Reducing constraints is thorny and intricate in institutional settings, unless you possess the power, of course. The desiderata of lowered constraints include responsive management, greater practitioner autonomy, creative work patterns, honest communication, and respect for the person of the clinician. Leaders must recognize that clinicians can be traumatized and that vicarious suffering is part of the work. Managers must strive to enhance the work experience to give workers more influence in policy decisions.

In attempting to increase supports and lower constraints, beware what has been labeled "false interventions" (Edelwich & Brodsky, 1980) that are handed out like candy on Halloween. When the staff becomes disgruntled and the workplace stale, managers are apt to run a 1-day workshop. Spirits are lifted for a few days or weeks, but little has materially changed. What all false interventions share in common is the premise that a person can deal with burnout once and for all through a single expedient. All of them attempt to disguise the omnipresent reality of occupational hazards with short-term fixes that, in actuality, fix nothing of the underlying causes in the long term (Edelwich & Brodsky, 1980). Treat the systemic roots, not only the acute symptoms.

Increasing supports and lowering constraints allow practitioners to work in high-demand institutional settings with severely and chronically ill patients. The research confirms collective experience: it's not the patients who drive us crazy; it's this place and its crazy administration.

SHALL I STAY OR SHALL I GO?

A courageous examination of your workplace's physical environment, social support, and administrative policies may lead to a decision that it cannot be fixed, not even measurably improved. The work environment is simply not tenable for you. You may decide to leave that workplace.

Following are two representative observations from workshop participants who came to such somber conclusions:

> "The self-care seminar helped me to realize that working in this particular university counseling center is a toxic work environment, at least currently, and is not likely to change in the near future. As a result, I will be going into full-time private practice after this semester ends. Probably not the response that you will get from many directors, but one that is right for me."

> "Your workshop helped me accept that there is really no way for me to remain in full-time practice at this time without compromising my emotional, mental, interpersonal, and spiritual well-being. So I have

scaled back my practice (about 30% so far) and am seriously considering closing it—at least temporarily."

Each colleague took brave actions in the best sense of self-care. Each colleague, at last contact, was eagerly pursuing alternatives—one in a different employment setting and the other in different work spheres—gardening, painting, and dance—"that float my heart."

A SELF-CARE VILLAGE IN A WORKAHOLIC WORLD

"Although we had been doing yoga twice a week in the office, this has fizzled and I need to revive it. I must admit that I worry how this is perceived by the administration . . . slackers in the counseling center. Should I care? This is a classic conflict in a productivity-minded work environment. My challenge now is how to best intervene in a systemic way in a university culture where workaholism and lack of value on self-care are relatively entrenched. I'd appreciate hearing any words of wisdom about how to create a systemic change in self-care."

Uh-oh. Words of wisdom? Hmmm. Well, certainly we can be supportive of our workshop participants' attempts to build self-care into the institutional ethos. And we are absolutely empathic. It frequently feels that we are only self-care spitting into a workaholic ocean. Workaholism is rewarded lavishly in most employment contexts, as we can guiltily attest. It is challenging enough to implement self-care in ourselves, but a Gordian knot to implement it into an entire institution.

On one level, self-care runs against the ingrained notion that "we are here for the clients," that "patients must come first." Understandably and rightly so. But the apparent paradox resolves itself as soon as one appreciates that psychotherapist self-care is a *critical prerequisite* for patient care.

Organizations frequently devalue supportive work practices, which are seen as self-indulgent in environments stressing productivity and efficiency. Further, individual practitioners are stigmatized as vulnerable if they accept support. Several surveys and a couple of interview studies have determined that psychotherapists may be vulnerable to poor levels of self-care because they perceive the expression of needing support as psychologically threatening. A psychotherapist is supposed to be "the strong one," right? (Canter, 1997). The psychotherapist's own fears of being a client (feeling out of control and, compared to colleagues, perhaps not coping well with high job stress) and the perceived cost of the support process itself discline individuals to create supportive environments (Walsh & Cormack, 1994).

What, then, can be done? Build a self-care village in a workaholic world.

First, pour the foundation by persistently advocating for self-care as a means of increasing productivity, enhancing outcomes, and promoting employee satisfaction and retention. As long as occupational stress is perceived as boosting productivity, there will be no compelling reason for organizations to even consider reducing or eliminating worksite stressors (Maslach & Goldberg, 1998). Self-care improves both practitioner health *and* patient outcomes—they are inseparable in our "business." Argue long and hard, at every opportunity in your institution, for psychotherapist self-care as improving the bottom line.

Next, erect the village's buildings by working with colleagues to challenge the pernicious beliefs that psychotherapists who seek support are weak and will be subtly punished (Walsh & Cormack, 1994). Daily we remind our clients that seeking psychological treatment is healthy and mature, but many in our profession do not apply the same lesson to themselves. Cultivate an ethos of staff support.

One interesting method is Me-Time (Maier & Van Rybroek, 1995). During this specifically scheduled period during the workday, distressed clinicians are encouraged to vent negative feelings that could potentially affect their work with patients. The combined forces of venting, group support, and peer feedback help relieve the distress and develop effective coping strategies (Miller, 1998).

Finally, top off the buildings' roofs by modeling self-care yourself and building it into the very structure of the operation. Put self-care on the agenda of each staff meeting. Track it as you would patient outcomes. Organize in-service activities or retreats on self-care. Include it in the annual staff evaluations. A creative colleague in one of our workshops wrote that

> "I brought back some of the ideas from those presentations and shared them with my staff. We held a retreat in January and focused on the issue of self-care. As a result, we have been drawing names each week and honoring a different staff member (kind of like giving them an extra birthday). This seems to have helped the morale."

SYSTEMS OF SELF-CARE

Self-care needs to be addressed at multiple levels: the individual practitioner, the physical environment, the organizational context, and the larger systems of the mental health professions. Before we conclude this chapter, we devote a couple of pages to these larger, systemic contexts.

Training Programs

We need to improve the psychological healthiness of our training programs. In one study of graduate students in psychology, 83% said their training program did not offer written materials on self-care (Munsey, 2006). Based on our teaching experience and the training literature, a horde of urgent corrections spring to mind, including:

- Select students for their interpersonal skills and self-development commitments in addition to their GREs and GPAs.
- Broaden the rubric of psychotherapy training to something like *developing or preparing psychotherapists* (after all, the term *training* that can connote a purely mechanical pursuit such as training seals to clap their flippers or training rats to run a maze; Bugental, 1987).
- Look at both the self and the system in training, as opposed to focusing on the "bad apple" of the impaired student (Forrest, Elman, Gizara, & Vacha-Haase, 1999; O'Connor, 2001).
- Undertake a program audit to determine how the training program is and is not incorporating humane values and self-care.
- Prepare psychotherapists who are, at once, technically competent *and* interpersonally capable.
- Recommend self-care for students enthusiastically.
- Increase the availability and affordability of personal therapy for students, such as maintaining lists of local practitioners offering reduced fees.
- Offer seminars addressing the occupational hazards of the profession and self-care methods.
- Model openness toward personal therapy and self-development by faculty and supervisors.
- Encourage research investigating psychotherapist self-care and development throughout the professional lifespan.

Most practitioners are simply unprepared by graduate programs for the emotional demands of practice. A conspiracy of silence surrounds practitioner distress and impairment. This omission encourages psychotherapists to distance themselves from their troubled colleagues and to think of them as a separate "not-like-me" group (O'Connor, 2001). This demonizing must stop, beginning with graduate training.

Licensing Boards

State licensing boards operate primarily to protect the public—a necessary and noble function—but some boards do not see a way to help practitioners in the process (O'Connor, 2001). Diversion and rehabilitation programs are effective in most cases, but some boards seem bent upon retribution. It's time to enlarge the mandate of licensing boards to protect the public by educating and rehabilitating practitioners.

Society is best served by strengthening a large cadre of well-trained, effective professionals available to serve the underserved. Individual practitioners, concerned laypersons, and professional associations must advocate for legislation that enlarges the mandate of licensing boards to assist, not just restrict, practitioners.

Mental Health Professions

Self-care should start at the top: the large professional organizations. Dozens of these associations in psychology, psychiatry, counseling, social work, mental health nursing, family therapy, and so on can propel the self-care movement. Here are a few prime examples of how leadership from the top might proceed:

- Assist practitioners in proactively seeking personal treatment (beyond programs for impaired colleagues).
- Organize Colleague Assistance Programs that offer education, referral, and rehabilitation (see also Chapter 5).
- Dispute publicly the notion that the norm of returning to therapy constitutes "failure."
- Require, as a part of accreditation, teaching modules on the emotional tolls of practice and concomitant self-care.
- Publish articles periodically, and hold convention sessions on practitioner self-care activities.
- Offer regular continuing education on the prevention of burnout and the implementation of self-care.
- Insert language into ethical codes about the centrality of self-care and the need for professional development.
- Reverse the trend that favors reactive treatment for impairment to one that favors proactive self-care for growth.

IN CLOSING

Environmental control—making the environment work for you, not against you—correlates highly with self-care effectiveness. It is ironic that psychotherapists who are typically adept at maintaining interpersonal boundaries frequently ignore the environmental practicalities that profoundly influence their satisfactions. Avoid the fundamental attribution error by harnessing the power of the environment to enhance your practice and yourself. The goal is not to survive but to flourish.

Self-care consists not simply of the internal or psychological factors of the psychotherapist, nor simply the external or situational factors. Instead, it is truly an interactional environment–person match in which the particulars of individual practitioners intertwine with the specifics of the work environment. The greater the gap, or misfit, between the job and person, the greater the likelihood of stress (Maslach & Goldberg, 1998). The greater the congruence, or fit, between job and person, the greater the rewards and satisfaction. And, being more human than otherwise, we psychotherapists have the capability to choose and remake our work environment.

SELF-CARE CHECKLIST

✓ Avoid falling prey to American individualism and the fundamental attribution error: Harness the power of your work environment to flourish.

✓ Conduct an environmental audit of your workspace for comfort and appeal.

✓ Improve your work environment by providing pleasure in your furniture, aesthetics in your decor, and replenishment in your cupboard.

✓ Increase sensory awareness: using vision, hearing, touch, and olfaction counterbalances the cognitive and affective work of psychotherapy.

✓ Take protective measures to ensure your safety and that of your practice environment.

✓ Give yourself time between patients, 10 minutes to breathe, relax, make notes, review notes, return calls, and process what has happened during the preceding 50 minutes.

✓ Determine whether your clinical talents and interpersonal interests are poorly invested in paperwork. If so, consider a computer, a clerical assistant, a billing service, or other alternatives.

✓ Delegate, defer, and simplify the business aspects of your clinical position.

✓ Build behavioral boundaries to temporarily separate yourself from the clinical world by means of routines and time.

✓ Increase supports and reduce constraints to keep high-demand institutional jobs bearable and rewarding.

✓ Search for ways to create greater freedom and independence in your work.

✓ Beware of false interventions and short-term fixes in dysfunctional institutions; treat the systemic roots, not just the acute symptoms.

✓ Create a self-care village in a workaholic world by advocating for self-care as a means of improving productivity and outcomes.

✓ Assist your colleagues and administrators in acknowledging the occupational hazards and in offering group support, Me-Time, and other replenishment opportunities.

✓ Cultivate a self-care ethos in clinical training by improving the selection of students, broadening the training goals, increasing the availability of personal therapy, modeling the commitment to personal development, and encouraging research on psychotherapist self-care.

✓ Begin self-care at the top: insist that your professional associations include self-care in their ethics, accreditation standards, publications, conferences, and continuing education.

RECOMMENDED READING

Guy, J. D., Brown, C. K., & Poelstra, P. L. (1992). Safety concerns and protective measures used by psychotherapists. *Professional Psychology: Research and Practice, 23*, 421–423.

Leiter, M. P., & Maslach, C. (2005). *Banishing burnout: Six strategies for improving your relationship with work.* San Francisco: Jossey-Bass.

Maslach, C., & Leiter, M. P. (1997). *The truth about burnout: How organizations cause personal stress and what to do about it.* San Francisco: Jossey-Bass.

O'Connor, M. F. (2001). On the etiology and effective management of professional distress and impairment among psychologists. *Professional Psychology: Research and Practice, 32*, 345–350.

CHAPTER 10

Undergoing Personal Therapy

An entire chapter on personal psychotherapy as self-care? You bet.

Personal treatment is, in many respects, the epicenter of the educational and self-care universe for psychotherapists (Norcross, 2005b). Our training, identity, health, and self-renewal revolve around the personal therapy experience. In their early classic *Public and Private Lives of Psychotherapists*, Henry and colleagues (1973, p. 14) conclude, "In sum, the accumulated evidence strongly suggests that individual psychotherapy not only serves as the focal point for professional training programs, but also functions as the symbolic core of professional identity in the mental health field."

By their behavior, practitioners embody this conclusion. Approximately three-quarters of mental health professionals have undergone personal psychotherapy, typically on several occasions. And, as we shall see, the benefits are overwhelmingly positive and multifaceted.

The relative importance attached to personal therapy varies systematically with one's own treatment history and theoretical orientation. Psychotherapists who have received personal treatment believe it is more important, while psychotherapists who have not think it is important but less so—96% versus 61% in one of our studies (Norcross et al., 1992). Psychoanalytic therapists have the highest rates of personal treatment (82–100%) and behavior therapists the lowest (44–66%) in the United States (Norcross & Guy, 2005). International studies (Orlinsky et al., 2005) reveal similar patterns: 92% of analytic/psychodynamic therapists and 92% of humanistic therapists from around the globe report having undergone personal therapy, whereas 60% of cognitive-behavioral therapists report doing so.

We, the authors, admit to a personal bias and even a potential conflict of interest here: about one-half of our psychotherapy patients are fellow mental health professionals. Lest it be thought that we are recruiting, we rush to reassure you that we both maintain part-time practices. It is a deep privilege to work with psychotherapists—in personal therapy, consultation, and workshops—and to assist them in navigating and nourishing their lives.

But we do not share their stories or cases here. There have been far too many inappropriate disclosures of confidential material in the literature already. We and our spouses have suffered the pain of learning that our privacy, our secrets, have been violated by those who promised confidentiality. Not coincidentally, fear of lapses in privacy and confidentiality emerges as a leading reason that seasoned practitioners do not return for personal therapy (e.g., Farber, 2000; Holzman, Searight, & Hughes, 1996). Following in the footsteps of our late friend Michael Mahoney (2003), we have come to regard confidentiality not only as a professional obligation but as a sacred commitment. Loose lips sink ships and beget mistrust of the enterprise.

From the beginning, Freud proposed that personal therapy was the deepest and most rigorous part of one's clinical education. In *Analysis Terminable and Interminable*, he (1937/1964, p. 246) rhetorically asked, "But where and how is the poor wretch to acquire the ideal qualification which he will need in this profession? The answer is in an analysis of himself, with which his preparation for his future activity begins."

At the same time, Freud was convinced of the value of ongoing personal therapy. Freud—and we—recommended that the clinician reinitiate personal treatment based on the recognition that practicing therapy continually exposes her to the impact of patients' psychopathology and on the need to know and utilize one's own responsiveness in conducting therapy. "Every analyst," Freud wrote (1937/1964, p. 249), "should periodically—at intervals of five years or so—submit himself to analysis once more, without feeling ashamed of taking this step. This would mean, then, that not only the therapeutic analysis of patients but his own analysis would change from a terminable to an interminable task."

In this chapter, we advance and amplify Freud's position in regard to self-care. The cumulative results argue that personal therapy is an emotionally vital and professionally nourishing experience central to the self-care of clinicians. The entire chapter is devoted to personal therapy as a prerequisite to conducting psychotherapy *and* as a corequisite of self-care over one's professional lifespan.

DEFINING OUR TERMS

In this chapter and in our research, *personal therapy* is a generic term encompassing psychological treatment of mental health professionals (and those in training) by means of various theoretical orientations and treatment formats (Norcross, 2005b). Personal therapy can thus refer to 12 sessions of group therapy for a graduate student, a year of couples therapy for a psychiatric resident, 3 years of intensive individual psychotherapy for a licensed psychologist, or ongoing 10-year treatment for a seasoned social worker. We reserve the term *training analysis* for the specific case of individual psychoanalysis required by a formal postgraduate psychoanalytic institute.

Personal therapy can be either voluntary or required. In most European countries, a specified number of hours of personal therapy is required in order to become accredited or licensed as a psychotherapist (Orlinsky et al., 2005). In the United States, by contrast, only psychoanalytic training institutes and a few graduate programs require a course of personal therapy.

GOALS OF PERSONAL THERAPY

Psychotherapists may seek personal therapy for personal reasons, for training/professional reasons, or for both reasons. Although oversimplified in a profession where the personal and the professional are nearly inseparable, the question does afford insight into psychotherapists' motivations. What are the goals in undergoing personal therapy?

In a word, personal. We reviewed five studies that asked psychotherapists their reasons for seeking personal therapy, and in all studies the majority (50–67%) indicated that they entered primarily for personal reasons (Norcross & Connor, 2005). When psychotherapists were asked to check their reasons for involvement in personal therapy, 60% checked personal growth, 56% checked personal problems, and 46% checked training (Orlinsky et al., 2005). Before, during, or after training, the results are clear: therapists largely enter psychotherapy to deal with "personal stuff."

Moreover, our presenting problems are, by and large, nearly identical to those of the educated populace seeking mental health services. Despite the enormous responsibilities of the profession, few psychotherapists identify the presenting problem or precipitant for their personal therapy as a problematic patient. In a couple of our early studies (Norcross & Prochaska, 1986b; Norcross, Prochaska, & DiClemente, 1986), involving hundreds of seasoned practitioners, only *one* psychologist identified the precipitant as a patient problem, in this case, a suicide attempt. The remaining 99% listed a nonpatient factor as the precipitant. In the context of a therapist's life-space, patient conflicts emerge as a moderate source of distress; extratherapy life problems are much more likely the reason for personal treatment. While we may be tempted to fantasize that seasoned psychologists are able to inoculate themselves against the ravages of life that beset their patients, the literature compellingly indicates otherwise (Norcross & Connor, 2005).

In this respect, let us cast the purposes of personal therapy in a systemic context. The primary goal of the psychotherapist's personal treatment is indeed personal, that is, to enhance the awareness, functioning, and life satisfaction of the person who, coincidentally, is a mental health professional. A secondary goal of personal treatment is to alter the nature of subsequent therapeutic work in ways that enhance its effectiveness. That is, personal treatment is designed both to enhance the personal functioning of the person and to improve her professional performance.

HOW PERSONAL THERAPY MAY ENHANCE CLINICAL EFFECTIVENESS

The mechanisms of securing these twin goals are as complex and individualized as the number of therapist–patients. Nonetheless, there are at least six recurrent themes in the literature relating to how the therapist's therapy is said to improve her clinical work (Norcross, Strausser-Kirtland, & Missar, 1988):

1. *Personal treatment improves the emotional and mental functioning of the psychotherapist: it makes the clinician's life less neurotic and more gratifying in a profession where one's personal health is an indispensable foundation.* Both common sense and the research literature demonstrate that therapist stress compromises professional functioning. Stressed, harried, dissatisfied therapists are not in a position to bring their best efforts to their work. If we fall apart, what is left for our clients?

2. *Personal treatment provides the therapist-patient with a more complete understanding of personal dynamics, interpersonal elicitations, and conflictual issues: the therapist will thereby conduct treatment with clearer perceptions, fewer contaminated reactions, and reduced countertransference potential.* Freud (1910/1957) famously wrote that "no psycho-analyst goes further than his own complexes and internal resistances permit."

3. *Personal treatment alleviates the emotional stresses and burdens inherent in the practice of psychotherapy: it enables practitioners to deal more successfully with the special problems imposed by the craft.* We itemized most of these special problems of the impossible profession in Chapter 3. Is there any kind of work in this world where the tools never get dulled, chipped, or broken (Lasky, 2005)?

4. *Personal treatment serves as a profound socialization experience: it establishes a sense of conviction about the validity of psychotherapy, demonstrates its transformational power in our own lives, and facilitates the internalization of the healer role.* It is sometimes asserted that what is most crucial about personal therapy is that clinicians have at least one experience of personal benefit, so that they acquire a sense of the potency of psychotherapy that can be communicated to their own patients. By this criterion, 85% of therapists acknowledge at least one such very positive experience—and some of those who have not yet had it might be expected to do so eventually (Orlinsky et al., 2005).

5. *Personal treatment places therapists in the role of the client: it thus sensitizes them to the interpersonal reactions and needs of their clients and increases respect for their patients' struggles.* Anyone who has ever suffered from a callous or insensitive remark from her personal therapist knows of what we speak. In fact, the most frequent lasting lessons practitioners take from their personal therapy concern the interpersonal relationships and dynamics of psychotherapy: the centrality of warmth, empathy, and the personal relationship; knowing what it feels like to be a patient; and the importance of transference and countertransference (Norcross, Strausser-Kirtland, & Missar, 1988; Norcross et al., 1992).

6. *Personal treatment provides a firsthand intensive opportunity to observe clinical methods: the therapist's therapist models interpersonal and technical skills.* Many are the times we have answered our patients with our therapist's words.

OUTCOMES OF PERSONAL THERAPY

Well, then, does undergoing personal therapy actually make a "significant" difference? Probably so. Below we briefly summarize the empirical evidence relating to the multitudinous outcomes of the psychotherapist's own psychotherapy. These outcomes encompass, inter alia, effects on subsequent therapy performance, self-reported outcomes, and impact on professional development (see Geller, Norcross, & Orlinsky, 2005, for detailed reviews).

The question of whether the practitioner who has undergone personal therapy can be empirically shown to be more effective than colleagues who have not received such therapy has been occasionally investigated. All of the early reviewers (e.g., Clark, 1986; Greenberg & Staller, 1981; Macran & Shapiro, 1998) concluded that there is no evidence that engaging in personal therapy is positively or negatively related to client outcome. In our recent review of this literature (Orlinsky et al., 2005), we echoed our colleagues' overwhelming laments about the poor quality of the studies to date.

Consequently, we must remember that studies on this matter conducted to date have suffered from the absence of large samples, controls, random assignment to personal therapy or nontherapy, and prospective designs. The net result is that we are left with interesting, retrospective looks at a complex interplay with little sensitivity and poor specificity. With so little and such insensitive research conducted in the past (and probably in the future) on the relationship between therapists' personal therapy and their subsequent outcomes with patients, the vital data will necessarily hail from psychotherapist research.

Moving from outcome to process studies, the existing evidence is more supportive. Early process studies (e.g., Wogan & Norcross, 1985) have found that the experience of personal therapy has several positive effects on the therapy relationship, specifically in facilitating empathic ability and decreasing one's dislike of patients. A review (Macran & Shapiro, 1998) of this small body of correlational studies was undertaken on the effects of personal treatment on the therapist's in-session behavior. The experience of personal therapy has been positively associated with the clinician's self-reported and rater-observed warmth, empathy, genuineness, awareness of countertransference, and increased emphasis on the therapeutic relationship. However, the research is again limited in the number of studies and the rigor of methodology.

While controlled experimental evidence is lacking on personal therapy, its desirability for psychotherapists is well established on other grounds. Across seven studies on the outcomes of personal treatment, therapist–patients find it helpful in 90%+ of the cases (Orlinsky et al., 2005). Although the studies ask the question in different ways, the self-reported outcomes are consistently positive. Even when accounting for cognitive dissonance and sanguine memories, the vast majority of therapists reported positive gains. Moreover, psychotherapists relate improvement in multiple areas: self-esteem, work functioning, social life, emotional expression, characterological conflicts, and symptom severity. The self-rated outcomes for improvement in behavior-symptoms, cognitive-insight, and emotions-relief are practically identical (Norcross, Strausser-Kirtland, & Missar, 1988), perhaps with symptom alleviation being slightly lower (Buckley, Karasu, & Charles, 1981).

Likewise, in the largest psychotherapist study conducted to date, Orlinsky and Rønnestad (2005) collected data on the personal therapy experiences of more than 4,000 therapists of diverse theoretical orientations in over a dozen countries. On self-report measures of consumer satisfaction, psychotherapists—arguably, the most discriminating consumers of psychotherapy one can imagine—positive outcomes predominate. Overall, 88% rated their personal benefit positively. Just 5% felt they received little personal benefit, and only 1% felt they had gotten nothing at all from their treatment.

At the same time, as with all psychotherapy, a small minority did report negative outcomes as a result of personal treatment. Across studies, the percentage of negative or harmful outcomes hovers between 1 and 5% (Norcross & Guy, 2005). In the international database, rates for unsatisfactory outcomes were generally between 3 and 7% (Orlinsky et al., 2005).

Another possible outcome of personal therapy is impact on professional development. In their pioneering study, Henry, Sims, and Spray (1971) asked their sample to evaluate the significance of various aspects of their training experience for their career. The most frequent training experiences recognized as important were field experience, personal therapy, and clinical supervision. Second only to practical experience, then, personal psychotherapy was cited by clinicians as the most important contributor to their professional development.

Similar results were found in the recent study of 4,000+ psychotherapists (Orlinsky & Rønnestad, 2005). Personal therapy consistently ranked among the top three sources of positive development, following direct patient contact and formal case supervision. Personal therapy clearly ranked above didactic experiences, such as taking courses and reading professional journals. Overall, more than three-quarters of psychotherapists across multiple studies found that their personal therapy had a strongly positive influence on their development as therapists, while fewer than 3% reported that it had a negative impact (Orlinsky et al., 2005).

Randomized clinical trials on the efficacy of psychologists' personal therapy have not been conducted and probably never will be; nonetheless, the available evidence on its personal and professional value is compelling. Fully 90% of psychologists who have undergone personal therapy report beneficial results across a range of outcomes, and over three-quarters relate that it had a strong positive influence on their development as psychotherapists. Further, the thousands of our peers participating in these studies indicate that the impact of their personal therapy is generally more formative than traditional coursework, which we rarely question as indispensable. The overwhelming bulk of evidence, with the exception of the inconclusive effects of personal therapy on subsequent patient outcomes, attests to its evidence-based position in the formation of psychotherapists (Norcross, 2005b).

SELF-CARE PRACTICES

Given the positive and pervasive outcomes of personal therapy for the practitioner, we recommend the following 10 self-care pursuits for your consideration.

Commence Personal Treatment at the Beginning of Your Career

Personal therapy's outcomes and impacts justify the widespread practice of undertaking extensive psychotherapy. Start the self-care early in your career.

Two of our master clinicians relate how they used their personal therapy from the beginning:

> "I was at an analytic institute, so I went to psychoanalysis three times a week. If there was anything that I was concerned about with a patient, I knew I could talk about it there and explore my feelings. I could explore if I was doing the right thing or something about my own experiences was coloring how I was reacting."

> "I did this [personal therapy] when I was in school, and I continued later in a lengthy treatment. It helps me to use my countertransference in a way that is helpful rather than destructive to the patient. When the patient talks about something that might resonate with my life, I don't get caught up in the issues that I have regarding that situation. I can stay focused on the issue as it occurred in the patient's life, and I can use the feelings that I have about that to energize the work I do with that patient."

Select Your Psychotherapist Carefully

Several of our studies have looked at the selection of the therapist's therapist to ascertain how it might best be done (e.g., Grunebaum, 1983; Norcross, Strausser, & Faltus, 1988). Therapist selection was predicated primarily on perceived competence, clinical experience, professional reputation, and interpersonal warmth. Six additional criteria were "somewhat important": openness; theoretical orientation; reputation for being a therapists' therapist; flexibility; not attributing everything to transference; and an active therapeutic style. By contrast, the research productivity of the potential psychotherapist was rated as a negligible factor in selection decisions. The latter finding should remind us that academic standing and clinical expertise are probably orthogonal dimensions.

What we have learned that may be useful in selecting therapists is to select a person capable of providing a personal relationship—one in which you feel affirmed, appreciated, and respected by another human being whom you like, appreciate, and respect. That this holds true for psychologically sophisticated patients, as it has been shown to be for more naive patients, corroborates the view that these factors are probably essential for effective psychological treatment, as Carl Rogers pointed out decades ago. What's more, negative effects of personal therapy are typically related to a poor therapeutic relationship (Orlinsky et al., 2005).

The growing availability of female, nonmedical, and nonpsychoanalytic psychotherapists now allow mental health professionals to be treated by members of their own gender, discipline, and orientation. We, among others (e.g., Ekstein & Wallerstein, 1972; Yalom, 2002), suggest that you carefully weigh the conflicting values of seeking personal treatment with a same-sex and like-minded psychotherapist. On the one hand, therapy with someone who belongs to the same school of thought can foster personal validation, interpersonal modeling, identity formation, and theoretical socialization. The best psychotherapeutic experience might be one that is more or less based on the same theoretical principles that the practitioner will eventually use. On the other hand, this matching can promote professional indoctrination and theoretical "inbreeding." The theoretical identification may slip into conversion, might discourage experimentation with different schools of thought, and might prevent the opening of minds. These are dialectical considerations for all psychologists seeking personal therapy, particularly for those in graduate training. Although students may have to sacrifice the certainty that accompanies orthodoxy, they may obtain something quite precious—a greater appreciation of the complexity and uncertainty underlying the therapeutic enterprise (Yalom, 2002).

Pursue Couple and Family Therapy as Well

This chapter has presumed so far individual therapy for the clinician, but we hasten to broaden the self-care perspective to couple and family therapy. The prevalence of couple and family therapy is lower than individual therapy: approximately 15% of psychotherapists receive couple therapy and 6% receive family therapy after receiving their degree (Guy, Poelstra, & Stark, 1988), compared to 50–60% securing individual therapy after receiving their degree. Nonetheless, many therapists have found it effective in ameliorating their family conflict or couple distress (Kaslow & Schulman, 1987)—or for growth work, not necessarily for psychopathology. We also recommend simultaneous or sequential systemic therapy for interpersonal conflicts and individual therapy for intrapsychic conflicts (insofar as we can separate them).

We are also enthusiastic promoters of family of origin work for the psychotherapist. All too often, our motives for becoming a psychotherapist are unexplained and unexplored. Simplistic self-care formulas operate like a band-aid in such circumstances; sophisticated self-care rests on understanding the deep familial roots of our calling (Guy, 1987). All therapists, we believe, need to examine their roles and scripts in their FOO (family of origin; Grosch & Olsen, 1994). Unconscious roles and expectations begin early; recall the saying that "most psychotherapists are born and the rest created by their families of origin." Imprints of families are played out in vocational choice, interpersonal relationships, and work environments. To some degree, we all repeat the themes of our families and the legacies of our childhood (Grosch & Olsen, 1994).

One of us (JCN), for example, discovered the early origins of becoming an integrative psychotherapist only in his personal therapy later in life. There was a profound but largely hidden influence of a parental legacy and ordinal position (Norcross, 2006). In some ways, I was integrative from the "get-go" and perhaps overdetermined by my family of origin. As the second of four children, my ordinal position (birth order) directed me to both mediate and rebel. Reliable adult observers concur that I would serve as the go-between for my brothers and serve as the bridge between my older domineering brother and my two younger siblings—a familiar pattern (or reconstruction) among psychotherapists in general (Dryden & Spurling, 1989; Henry et al., 1971).

Research, practice, and experience converge in our recommending family of origin work for many psychotherapists. We all need to learn the messages we received, and the roles we played, in our families of origin. These past experiences are probably replicated in our career decisions and in our current work. As Faulkner reminds us, "The past is never dead. It's not even past."

Embrace the Wounded Healer Inside

The notion that the psychotherapist's pain and disorder may sometimes be advantageous in clinical work is deeply rooted in both Eastern philosophies and in classical mythology. In Greek myths, for example, the centaur Chiron was a mortally wounded healer who taught humans the art of medicine. From his wounds came knowledge and skills that helped others. The mythical figure Asklepios (or Aesculapius) was, in turn, raised by Chiron. Asklepios developed mighty healing powers despite the fact that he suffered from a personal wound that would not heal (Mahoney, 2003). When properly treated, therapist wounds can strengthen and enrich work with clients.

What is wounded about the wounded healer is a matter of interpretation. In some cultures, *wounded* means little more than a veteran of life experiences. In some spiritual cultures, love is described as a permanently open wound—an ever flowing aperture on life. In industrialized cultures, *wounded* tends to have more negative connotations, where "vulnerability" (literally, the capacity to be wounded) is equated with illness and disorder (Mahoney, 2003). We mean it as sensitive, experienced, "been there" empathy; *wounded* denotes to us vulnerable and wise in a positive sense. Where wound is, there is also genius.

Confront Your Resistance about Pursuing Personal Therapy

In an early article, Arthur Burton (1972) summarized major resistances that serve as reasons for healers not entering personal therapy. One resistance is that psychotherapists are ever fearful of personal regression and giving up power to another. The therapist's self-image and narcissism are such that she feels her self-knowledge and humanity are just a shade above that of other healers. Another resistance to personal psychotherapy is shame—"a kind of damage that is done to a healer when he is forced to become a fellow sufferer of those he regularly treats, that is so subtle and intangible as to defy description" (Burton, 1972, p. 100).

At least five studies have taken the interesting twist of asking mental health professionals for their reasons in not seeking personal therapy (Norcross & Connor, 2005). While there are some differences evident in the results across studies, probably owing to methodological and sampling disparities, there is a robust consistency in the rationale for not undergoing personal therapy. These are confidentiality concerns, financial expenses, exposure fears, self-sufficiency desires, time constraints, and difficulties in locating a good enough therapist outside of their immediate social and professional network. A sizable percentage also note that they did not pursue personal treatment because other means proved effective in dealing with the inevitable burdens of life (and practicing psychotherapy).

To be sure, these are "good reasons" for not pursuing psychotherapy; yet, we cannot help but wonder whether these are convenient excuses for deeper resistances articulated by Burton (1972) and earlier by Freud (1937/1964). Many of us are blocked by the shame, by the difficulty in accepting the patient role. We are threatened by "needing help"; we desire to be self-reliant and close to perfect, not like "one of our patients." In fact, these are the very identity conflicts and narcissistic wounds with which psychotherapists are likely to struggle in personal therapy.

We hark back to the powerful defenses against awareness among our mental health colleagues. Two published examples jump out at us: a psychiatrist in practice for 27 years failing to recognize her own anxiety attack (Gartrell, 2004) and a psychologist-researcher, an expert on bipolar disorder, not recognizing her own bipolar disorder (Jamison, 1997). We are heartened when therapists write honestly and courageously about their own afflictions. Thousands more transpire yearly without being published.

Please examine closely your own resistances if you decide not to pursue personal therapy. There are alternatives to personal therapy, of course, but we recommend at a minimum that you permit a peer to take an independent, external look into your functioning.

Supplement Psychotherapy with Self-Analysis

Just as we remind our patients, psychotherapy must be complemented with self-analysis. We can strengthen and extend therapeutic analysis with our self-analysis.

Our clinical training is built upon the belief that when the self-understanding of the practitioner is ignored our clinical competence will be compromised and our personal lives will remain unfulfilled (Goldberg, 1993). Freud regarded self-examination to be indispensable and recommended that the psychotherapist continue a regular self-analysis after the practitioner's personal analysis was complete. Freud took his own medicine in this regard: he religiously attended to his own self-analysis the last hour of each day (Jones, 1955).

We are unaware of any hard statistics on the prevalence of self-analysis, but most seasoned psychotherapists state that such self-examination is a necessary part of effective practice, and they partake of it (Goldberg, 1992). Of course, there is the perennial problem in self-therapy of the dual relationship with your client!

One of the master clinicians we interviewed for this book told us:

"I work on my own dreams once a week for about 2 hours. What I do is work on my dreams, and then I apply my dream work to things that are bothering the hell out of me. If one patient is talking about killing himself, then I apply my dream work to that particular worry, and so whatever I get from my dreams I apply to what I'm going to do about that particular patient."

Self-analysis is highly effective in some cases, and in others the therapist may have a fool for a patient (Chessick, 1990). Self-analysis is surely an elusive and potentially deceptive task. It is a poorly understood but profound commitment to self-discovery. "The opportunity to deal with our deeply buried sense of despair about our human limitations enables us to live more legitimately as purposive people and to develop a courageous and creative consciousness of human possibility" (Goldberg, 1993, p. 161). Remember: you are the one patient that *never* leaves your practice.

Return to Personal Therapy Periodically

As a rule, psychotherapists pursue personal treatment on more than one occasion. Across studies, the number of discrete episodes averages between 1.8 and 3.0. In one of our studies (Norcross et al., 2005), 32% of psychologists sought personal therapy once, 32% sought therapy twice,

22% three times, and the remaining 14% sought therapy on four or more occasions.

A pernicious myth persists that most mental health professionals do not need personal therapy once they are in practice; however, the evidence rebuts any such illusion. Most seasoned clinicians do in fact utilize the very services they provide. About half of seasoned mental health professionals returned to personal therapy (range = 43–62%) following completion of formal training or the terminal degree (Norcross & Guy, 2005). Psychotherapists seeking personal treatment repeatedly during their careers supports the conclusion that it is widely perceived not only as an essential part of the formative training phase but also as an important component in the practitioner's ongoing maturation and regenerative development.

The firsthand accounts of therapist-patients make it compellingly clear that they seek different therapeutic goals at different seasons of their lives. In discussing his own odyssey of personal therapy over a 45-year career, Irv Yalom (2002, p. 42) pointedly observed: "I entered therapy *at many different stages of my life.* Despite an excellent and intensive course at the onset of one's career, an entirely different set of issues may arrive at different junctures of the life cycle."

What's more, a return to personal therapy for self-care allows the practitioner to address the underlying psychodynamics and vulnerabilities to particular stressors. Personal therapy later in life permits us to understand why we are not coping with a particular stressor and then responsively tailor self-care (House, 1995). It is challenging and lifelong work to decipher—and then integrate—our deepest pathologies and difficulties.

Obtain an Annual Satisfaction Checkup

Instead of, or in addition to, a return to personal therapy, we recommend an annual satisfaction checkup with a professional mentor or former therapist. Talk honestly to her about your aspirations, disappointments, fears, and joys. Ask for an assessment of your overall well-being. This annual ritual will help you track your progress in the journey of life.

Encourage Personal Therapy in the Profession

If we are to take personal therapy seriously as self-care, then we all need to support it throughout the professional lifespan, starting in graduate training. Personal therapy should occupy its rightful throne in the training enterprise as one empirically supported path toward self-development. Specifically, we hope that (Norcross, 2005b):

- Graduate programs in mental health will select students for their interpersonal skills and self-development interests in addition to their college grades and test scores.
- Descriptions of graduate programs will enthusiastically recommend personal treatment for their trainees.
- Training programs will increase the availability of personal therapy for their students, such as maintaining lists of local practitioners offering reduced fees.
- Class meetings will discuss the research on psychologists' personal therapy, emphasizing the impressively consistent reports of its multiple benefits and infrequent negative outcomes.
- Professors will model openness to personal therapy and self-development not as a singular event but as a continuous lifelong process.
- Researchers will investigate the moderators and mediators of effective personal psychotherapy as well as effective practices in conducting treatment with fellow mental health professionals.
- Local and state psychological associations will assist practitioners in proactively seeking personal treatment (beyond programs for impaired psychologists) and will publicly dispute the notion that the norm of returning to therapy constitutes "failure."
- Practitioners will, perhaps "at intervals of 5 years or so," submit themselves to psychotherapy once more—without "feeling ashamed."
- Professional organizations will advance the cause of personal therapy.

Regard as One Form of Self-Development

Our maxim of matching self-care to the unique needs of the individual practitioner would be violated by insisting on a single method for all. As enthusiastic as we are in our endorsement of personal therapy, we recognize that it is only one form of self-development. It is not *either* personal therapy or *nothing*; it is personal therapy *plus* the restorative self-care strategies covered elsewhere in this book.

We view personal therapy as one component of ongoing development and continuing education. Accordingly, we recommend a variety of individually tailored personal development exercises and other life-enhancing activities. These might include the creative arts, formal religious training, Buddhist retreats, meditation seminars, dream work, or self-help groups. All of these roads can lead to the same destination: enhanced personal functioning and professional performance of the person of the psychotherapist.

IN CLOSING

One can reasonably inquire: If you trust what you do with clients, why not do it with yourself? And, if you trust what you do with yourself, why not do it with your clients? (Mahrer, 2000). Use what you know about psychotherapy for and by yourself. Let us heed our own evidence, and let us practice what we preach about the marvels and mysteries of psychotherapy.

Here we encounter another concrete manifestation of the complex interweaving of personal dynamics and self-care. We must learn what motivates us to become therapists, learn what makes us run (excessively). Then we can develop a personalized regimen of self-care that speaks to our particular needs. We cannot mindlessly prescribe a mechanized regimen of self-care methods, no matter how effective. Personal therapy, in this sense, fuels and informs a lifetime of effective self-care.

We conclude with the words of one of our cherished colleagues, Laura Brown (2005, p. 956). She writes, "I will be in and out of therapy for the rest of my life, not because I see myself as especially wounded (I am at worst terrifically neurotic in an anxious, obsessive–compulsive sort of way), but because my work requires this of me, and I have learned to like this requirement."

SELF-CARE CHECKLIST

✓ Heed the evidence: personal therapy is an emotionally vital and professionally nourishing experience central to self-care.

✓ Give yourself 50 minutes of time every few weeks in a holding environment; practice what you preach about the value of psychotherapy!

✓ Confront your resistances for not pursuing personal therapy. Are these "good reasons"—or convenient rationalizations to avoid accepting the patient role?

✓ Take seriously Freud's recommendation that every therapist should periodically—at intervals of 5 years or so—reenter psychotherapy *without shame* as a form of continued education. Do you heed his sage advice? Do you struggle with the shame?

✓ Beware the illusion that mental health professionals do not experience a need for personal therapy once they are in practice. More than half of psychotherapists do receive personal treatment following completion of formal training.

✓ Seek family therapy and family of origin work as well; do not limit yourself to individual therapy.

✓ Supplement personal therapy with regular self-analysis.

✓ Consider an annual satisfaction checkup with a valued mentor, trusted colleague, or former therapist.

✓ Pursue other personal development activities in addition to personal therapy. These might include the creative arts, Buddhist training, meditation seminars, dream work, or self-help groups.

RECOMMENDED READING

Freud, S. (1964). Analysis terminable and interminable. In J. Strachey (Ed. and Trans.), *The standard edition of the complete psychological works of Sigmund Freud* (Vol. 23). London: Hogarth Press. (Original work published 1937)

Geller, J. D., Norcross, J. C., & Orlinsky, D. E. (Eds.). (2005). *The psychotherapist's own psychotherapy: Patient and clinician perspectives.* New York: Oxford University Press.

Guy, J. D., Poelstra, P. L., & Stark, M. J. (1988). Personal therapy for psychotherapists before and after entering professional practice: A national survey of factors related to its utilization. *Professional Psychology: Research and Practice, 19,* 474–476.

Norcross, J. C. (2005). The psychotherapist's own psychotherapy: Educating and developing psychologists. *American Psychologist, 60,* 840–850.

Yalom, I. (2002). *The gift of therapy: An open letter to a new generation of therapists and their patients.* New York: HarperCollins.

CHAPTER 11

Cultivating Spirituality and Mission

This was our most difficult chapter to write. Writing on the topic of spirituality and particularly religion is a perilous task, since the chances of offending the reader or being misunderstood are so great. In fact, we seriously considered dropping this chapter altogether. Obviously, we did not, but our concerns about how it will be received still remain.

We are convinced that spirituality is an indispensable source of strength and meaning for the psychotherapist. Too few books have addressed the transcendent aspects of psychotherapy, the role of the spiritual dimension in practice, and the therapist's vocational calling. While this chapter is certainly not intended to be an evangelistic plea for religious conversion or devotion, we do wish to provoke you to evaluate the sources of meaning and fulfillment in your own life. They must provide sustenance if you are to enjoy a long, satisfying, successful career as a psychotherapist.

The calling to be a clinician almost invariably involves a spiritual quest, or what Maslow (1971) characterized as a sense of mission. At the end of a long and grueling day of seeing patients, we might experience considerable difficulty in recalling what that mission is, but we do recognize it most of the time. The self-care imperative is to resonate or tap into that abiding mission, spirituality, or social interest. Something greater than ourselves, a transcendental endeavor. It can be a traditional religion, a new-age spirituality, or an ecumenical mission, but it renews and replenishes us. Indeed, the term *spirituality* derives from the Latin *spiritus*, meaning "breath of life."

We noted in Chapter 5 that nurturing relationships are one of the best predictors of life satisfaction or happiness (Myers, 2000). The other key predictor is the person's faith, which encompasses social support, purpose, and hope. Simply stated, the two best predictors of life satisfaction for people later in life are health and religiousness/spirituality (Okun & Stock, 1987).

A religious/spiritual commitment is also positively associated with physical health. A review of 200+ studies found that approximately 75% demonstrate a modest benefit for religious/spiritual commitment (Matthews et al., 1998). In healthy participants, a strong, consistent, and prospective reduction in mortality risk is found among church or service attenders. The reduction is approximately 25% after adjusting for confounders. Religion or spirituality protects against cardiovascular disease, largely mediated by the healthy lifestyle it encourages (Powell, Shahabi, & Thoreson, 2003).

We want to acknowledge at the outset that this chapter is influenced by the fact that we are both spiritual/religious individuals: one of us is devoutly religious in the Christian tradition; the other is devoutly spiritual in an eclectic mix of Protestantism and Judaism. Our personal faith provides an important sense of calling in our work as psychotherapists as well as meaning in our lives that is independent of our professional role.

Having said that, we are polytheists when it comes to psychotherapist self-care. Some of you will have found other sources of purpose and fulfillment that are not religious in nature. Others will have found meaning in a sense of spirituality or transcendence that is different from our own. We do not prescribe any particular form of "meaning making." Instead, we advocate for your personal (re)discovery of meaning and mission and your evaluation of them in your life and work.

The religious commitments of psychotherapists are more complex than suggested by the simple distinction between secular and religious. A study of roughly 1,000 psychotherapists from around the globe indicated that 51% of us can be characterized by a pattern of personal spirituality, 27% as religious spirituality, and only 21% a pattern of secular morality (Smith & Orlinsky, 2004). It is true that psychotherapists are less conventionally religious than the population in terms of formal organization and church attendance (e.g., Ragan, Malony, & Beit-Hallahmi, 1980), but we are quite a spiritual lot.

Such studies powerfully remind us that spirituality comes in many guises and that, in this book, we should avoid a single theocentric perspective. Some therapists find more comfort in an organized religion and a particular faith. Others find their mission in a broader belief system that transcends the demands and differences of specific religious groups. Still others find themselves and their vocations in nature or mysticism. All end up as spiritual beings, loved and valued by a spirit/nature with many names and manifestations. Our aim in this chapter is to stimulate you to capitalize on spirituality and mission as part of your self-care.

SPIRITUALITY AT THE OFFICE

The transcendent or spiritual aspects of psychotherapeutic practice are nearly ineffable. They almost defy description. The art of our work touches and invokes a spiritual dimension, and the energy and meaning that exist in this dimension hold great potential for empowering our life and practice (Grusky, 1987). Below we consider four pragmatic manifestations of spirituality at the office: our career as calling; care for others; commitment to growth; and spirituality in clinical practice.

Career as Calling

"Why did you become a psychotherapist?" We have all been asked (and challenged) about our career choice. Our vocational explanations bring an assortment of reactions from people, one of which is admiration. Many individuals decide that we must be special people to provide such caring and support on a daily basis—"I don't know how you listen to that stuff all day." Despite our realization that we are quite mortal and ordinary folks, there is a part of us that recognizes that we are indeed "different" and that we pursue a career for which most are not well suited. It *does* take a certain kind of individual to be a psychotherapist.

As psychotherapists, we know that we are not "special" in terms of personal worth, but we do recognize that we occupy a unique role in society. As spiritual descendants of the archetypal healer, we join a long line of special caregivers such as the witch doctor, wizard, priest, and family doctor. The position of the shaman has always been held in both honor and fear. The shaman's work is regarded as essential by the community, and yet his or her powers are shrouded in mystery. As a "wounded healer," the shaman's own pain gives insight and empathy into the suffering of others. His or her ability to overcome personal affliction gives evidence of power and authority over the forces that create suffering. Psychotherapists share in this tradition of healers, and their own pain informs their work with others. We are sojourners who join our clients in facing life's struggles together.

As we discussed in Chapters 2 and 3, psychotherapists select this career for reasons other than simply personal suitability. The desires to relieve distress and promote growth in others are primary motivators

(Guy et al., 1989). Quite simply, psychotherapists find it very satisfying to assist in psychic "healing." This healing process involves participating in an intense relationship. Rather than setting a broken bone and watching it heal, as would a physician, the psychotherapist participates in the healing process more directly, more personally. Indeed, she as a person is often the curative force. Becoming a part of another person's healing is a special privilege deeply appreciated by most psychotherapists; it allows us to transcend our own being and participate in a greater calling.

Vocation is more than simply performing a job, or paid employment; rather, it links who a person is to what a person does. Integrating vocation with psychotherapy brings deep satisfaction and enriched meaning to psychotherapy. One of our preeminent satisfactions is the ability to integrate vocation with our identity (Tieman, 1987)—what we do with who we are.

In Maslow's (1971, p. 291) pioneering work on self-actualizers, he found that "all such people are devoted to some task, call, vocation, beloved work (outside themselves)." Self-actualizers are, without exception, involved in a cause outside of their own skin. Their devotion and dedication are so marked that one can fairly use the old words *vocation, calling,* or *mission* to describe their passionate feeling for the "work." Further, Maslow (1971, p. 296) found that "the tasks to which they are dedicated seem to be interpretable as embodiments or incarnations of intrinsic values (rather than as a means to ends outside the work itself, and rather than as functionally autonomous). The tasks are loved (and introjected) BECAUSE they embody these values. That is, ultimately it is the values that are loved rather than just the job as such."

Mission is a distinguishing feature of self-actualizers and, we are convinced, the best of psychotherapists. Many psychotherapists feel called to the career—not simply out of family of origin experiences that created "natural-born healers," but as expressions of a deep sense of intrinsic value, something larger than themselves. Their calling, their mission, is something that "sets their hair on fire."

We are reminded of the refrain from one of our favorite inspirational hymns, "We Are Called": "We are called to act with justice, we are called to love tenderly, we are called to serve one another, to walk humbly with God." The song is riveting with a blaring organ and enthusiastic singers. It need not invoke a higher deity to convey its impact: we are called to a healing mission, to a sacred vocation.

Care for Others

Conducting psychotherapy involves the heart and soul of the practitioner. We bring not only an assortment of skills and techniques to the task but also our essential personhood to the encounter. Technical expertise is rarely sufficient to encourage growth in others. As Carl Rogers established decades ago, effective psychotherapists communicate a spirit of hope, vitality, and optimism that pervades the relationship.

Psychotherapists possess an enduring care and concern for others. They enjoy people, and they are able to appreciate the best qualities of the human spirit. Their capacity to love and appreciate their clients serves as a "life force" for their work. This is not a contrived clinical technique. Rather, it is an attitude of the heart that motivates the clinician to enter this profession, and it continues to provide fulfillment sufficient to cause the psychotherapist to remain in this career.

Intimate contact with patients is accompanied by a sense of awe and wonder at the human spirit. Spirituality (and religion) helps us to redis-cover or reawaken the awe of human existence. We become childlike—wow!—the wonder, the mystery, the splendor (Schneider, 2004).

Psychotherapists with strong religious or spiritual convictions have less difficulty in helping clients pull hope out of their hell. Our late friend Michael Mahoney (2003) was fond of saying that therapists are ex-pected to pull hope out of clients' hellish experiences—tragedy, heartless-ness, insensitivity, and violations of human decency. Therapists are socially sanctioned protectors of hope. "The therapists who lacks a hope-protecting philosophy of life may be particularly vulnerable to the chal-lenges presented by the 'hope from hell' paradox" (Mahoney, 2003, p. 197).

Commitment to Growth

To maintain our genuine caring and to pull hope from hell, psychothera-pists must be an optimistic cadre. They believe in the potential for signifi-cant growth and change in their clients—and themselves. They have tre-mendous respect for the resilience and tenacity of the human personality. Their optimism about the possibility of emotional growth usually pre-ceded their vocational choice, but this optimism was later confirmed by their personal therapy experiences (see Chapter 10) and strengthened by positive treatment outcomes.

Therapists exposed to trauma (that is, all of us) are confronted with spiritual challenges. Our basic faith in goodness is confronted with every case of inhumane cruelty. We confront daily our own sense of meaning and hope. Ironically, practitioners treating more abuse survivors report more existentially and spiritually satisfying lives than those with less expo-sure to trauma clients (Brady et al., 1999). They have a heightened empha-sis on meaning and hope. Perhaps purified by fire, therapists come out stronger and more resilient.

Spirituality begets optimism, be it here on this earthly plane or else-where in a cosmic paradise. Because they are faithful to the probability of growth, psychotherapists commit themselves to the healing process despite the hellish experiences. They bring all of their expertise and experi-ence to the task of promoting this growth. This partnership is anchored to the beliefs that the client can improve, the process of psychotherapy works, and the outcome will make all of the effort worthwhile.

Here's how one of our master clinicians described the benefits of his sense of spirituality:

> "It helps put things in perspective. I can get real involved in what's happening right here and right now. It helps me realize things are going to turn out well in the end even if they do not turn out well in the moment. Sometimes it's formal things like going to church, read-ing spiritual books, or praying everyday and reading the Bible. Some-times it's more free-form, like taking a walk in nature. My favorite is old gospel hymns, because they bring my spirits back."

The commitment to growth applies equally to the practitioner her-self. Psychotherapy as a career allows one to feel both agentic and com-munal, to feel an enhanced sense of identity and intimacy, to work in the service of self and others. This is a powerful motivator in simulta-neously advancing two causes in one profession (Farber & Norcross, 2005).

Spirituality in Clinical Practice

Calls for a renewed dialogue on spirituality and religion in psychotherapy reflect an increasing willingness for psychotherapists to examine the value of religious beliefs in their own lives as well as those of their clients (Jones, 1994). With a few exceptions, our master clinicians found renew-ing their sense of spirituality and mission to be a useful means of coping with occupational distress. An appreciation for the transcendent spiritual dimension of human existence is a constant source of meaning for many psychotherapists.

Much of what we believe and do as healing practitioners emanates from an implicit worldview or personal philosophy. Worth of the individ-ual and the potential for change are two exemplars. Perhaps the worth of the individual is based on respect for the human spirit, viewing it as pre-eminently valuable in and of itself as it joins with the life force of other human spirits. Or perhaps the human soul is seen as a participant in a larger spiritual force existing in all of nature or perhaps worthy of dignity and respect because it reflects God's image. Regardless of the particular view taken, most psychotherapists recognize that individuals possess worth and dignity in part because they belong to a force that transcends their own existence. Similarly, the therapist's belief in the potential for change is rooted in a spiritual worldview that believes people are drawn toward wholeness. Humans possess within themselves the potential for growth as well as destruction.

These are but a few examples of how a sense of spirituality can enhance our self-care. We are renewed in participating in the process of healing with patients. There is a sense in which the psychotherapist joins with the soul of the client, the forces of nature, and the very God of creation as she participates in the restoration of the client. Psychotherapy involves a profound "re-creating." The practitioner who sees herself participating in the meaningful restoration of another human being is filled with a sense of wonder and awe.

It becomes an honor and privilege to be included in the healing process. This phenomenon is described by one of our master clinicians:

> "I feel that my work is an act of worship. I believe that God uses me to help relieve human suffering and to bring wholeness to my clients. It's not unusual for them to become more religious during treatment. We sense God's hand at work in their lives. I feel that God has equipped me for this work. I'd be unhappy doing anything else."

An appreciation for the spirituality of clinical practice impacts how we approach our daily work. Those of us who believe that we are merely participants in clients' growth resist assuming ultimate responsibility for treatment progress; we do not believe we alone will determine eventual success. Instead, we recognize that we join with a Supreme Being or transcendent force that facilitates personality growth; we are instruments of healing but not the source of wholeness.

This worldview allows the practitioner to call on nature, God, or transcendent forces directly for assistance and encouragement. We can invoke the powers of the life force in nature or a tendency toward self-actualization within the client to supplement our ministrations. Personal prayer can offer comfort for the psychotherapist who feels overwhelmed or alone with the challenges of clinical practice (Galanter, Larson, & Rubenstone, 1991). The point we wish to make is that most psychotherapists find reassurance in recognizing that forces beyond their own ability are at work in the process of psychotherapy.

An appreciation for the spiritual within psychotherapy will also influence how practitioners approach terminations with clients. A trust in the personal responsibility of the client and the transcendent force that influences her spirit will allow the dedicated psychotherapist to let go of the client at the appropriate moment. Treatment must end, and eventually contact will cease. There is considerable comfort in remembering that growth will likely continue. Not only have patients internalized the resources provided by the therapist, but they have access to other resources beyond, including spiritual and self-actualizing forces.

The potential for career dissatisfaction and eventual burnout can be substantially reduced by conceptualizing our role as part of a larger transcendent scheme. Some researchers have found this to indeed be the case (e.g., Leighton & Royce, 1984). Those of us able to put work in this perspective, surrendering ultimate responsibility for clients and yet valuing the privilege of participating in their growth, will most likely find lasting meaning in our careers. We will know how and when to set aside the professional role and relax. Attaining inner peace through the pursuit of meaning in life is a highly rated means of coping with the pressures of clinical work (Medeiros & Prochaska, 1988).

Of course, psychotherapists are not to impose their spiritual beliefs or values onto clients. We must be mindful of professional ethics, especially when the client's religious views or commitments differ from those of the psychotherapist. This ethical proscription and the concomitant respect for the autonomy of the patient do not mean, however, that spirituality is out of bounds in clinical work. Far from it.

SPIRITUALITY OUTSIDE THE OFFICE

Patients can drain us, not simply of emotional resources, but also of deep faith. We have all felt like our lightbulb might go out, the well might run dry, or our energy become depleted (and a dozen other metaphors). Spirituality outside the office can renew us inside the office and, more fundamentally, replenish our personhood. Here are four paths advocated by the empirical research, clinical experience, and our own lives.

Pursuing Ultimate Questions

The psychotherapist confronts on a daily basis the ultimate questions of human existence, such as the meaning of life and the eventuality of death. These existential issues invariably touch on the spiritual needs of the clinician. And most will adopt a perspective that allows for the uniquely spiritual aspects in the human personality and the ongoing process of emotional growth (Shafranske & Malony, 1990).

As chronic "meaning makers," psychotherapists are determined to understand their place in this life. Like other curious, intelligent people, this may lead them to pursue formal or informal studies of theology, philosophy, science, or literature. It may also motivate them to travel widely, enriching their appreciation for the human condition through cross-cultural experiences. The desire to find meaning is reflected in their very career choice; it reflects and reinforces a lifelong commitment to understanding the "big picture."

It is important to remind ourselves that the practice of psychotherapy does not, in and of itself, provide ultimate meaning in our lives. It can provide great satisfaction and pleasure, but it does not provide the sole purpose for existence. This may seem obvious, but as we discussed in earlier chapters, the practice of psychotherapy has a pernicious tendency to envelop our lives—depleting our inner resources, preoccupying our mental life, and dominating consciousness. If we are not careful, our careers can become the exclusive source of meaning, thereby creating an unhealthy situation in which the practice of psychotherapy becomes the primary source of nurturance for the therapist. This is the road to burnout.

Ultimate meaning in life must be found outside the work of the psychotherapist. For some, relationships with loved ones and friends will satisfy this need. The love of a partner, the connection with children, and/or the affection of friends provide an intricate quiltwork of human relationships that fill us. For others, the meaning will be found elsewhere, such as in pursuing personal spirituality. The take-home message is to find it, and not exclusively in our careers.

Becoming a Citizen-Therapist

Participation in a broader community can generate meaning in the life of the psychotherapist. We can tackle the larger social, economic, and political issues of the day through social activism. We cannot be content to rant and rave at the morning's newspaper headlines or evening television newscasts, but rather should demonstrate a behavioral commitment to genuine changes in society. Citizen–therapists actually do something about it.

Tikkun (also *tikkun olam*) is a Hebrew term for healing or repairing the world. *Tikkun* is an important mission in Judaism and is often used to explain the Jewish concept of social justice. What is your *tikkun*?

Examples we have encountered:

- Transforming a poor community into a bastion of the middle class
- Giving marriage education away
- Enhancing women's rights
- Teaching conflict resolution skills
- Working with disaster victims
- Taking the fight to Capitol Hill
- Lobbying for universal health care
- Reducing community violence
- Correcting gender inequities
- Fighting against racism
- Battling on behalf of the environment and mother earth

These are personal as well as professional causes, and they call for responses as responsible citizens.

A personal case in point: One of us (JDG) directs a nonprofit institute devoted to providing psychological and spiritual support to humanitarian relief and development personnel worldwide. The institute has provided thousands of hours of training, consulting, and services to more than 2,000 individuals from over 50 countries (see *www.headington-institute.org* for details). This is our *tikkun*, our mission.

Social responsibility expressed in social activism is part of a spiritual mission. This serves as an outlet for frustration, binds anxiety, and focuses frustrated energies (Miller, 1998). Provided, of course, that the activism does not become an obsessional, dysfunctional "crusade."

Certain professional disciplines and theoretical orientations tend to gravitate toward distinctive missions. Social workers, as a rule, are trained in and committed to social welfare, justice, and community service. Staff members of women's resource centers are heavily invested in enhancing women's rights and self-determination. Clinicians working in disenfranchised urban centers are committed to the eradication of poverty, racism, and inequitable distribution of wealth. All are citizen-therapists expressing their mission, their *tikkun*, through social activism.

Integrating Religion and Spirituality into Your Personal Life

There is minimal integration of spiritual or religious content into clinical training and supervision (Hage, 2006). The topic is rarely broached. There is even less integration of spiritual/religious concerns into our personal lives during clinical training. It is almost never addressed in a systematic matter.

Outside of formal training, psychotherapists learn on their own to integrate spirituality and religion, as they experience it, into their lives. This process is part of a therapeutic underground—what every practitioners knows and practices but is rarely recorded in the professional literature.

One method we have used in our workshops to help practitioners renew their connection to spirituality is to ask them to take 10–15 minutes to write a stream of consciousness letter to God, Nature, Spirit, or a higher power. Their products are impressive—especially for the two of us, who are skeptical of gimmicky techniques—and contain some amazing realizations. The letters are too private to share here, as we did not ask permission to share their content. Nonetheless, we recommend this powerful method to reconnect with something limitless and larger. Many practitioners feel a peaceful calm and an overwhelming sense of unbounded possibilities after giving the method a try.

In the words of one workshop participant:

"Your workshop encouraged me to become serious about doing things that are important to my soul, as I am much more than just a clinician. I think that people in all professions should be encouraged to grow beyond their professional identity."

As with all broad self-care strategies, practitioners will select those specific methods that resonate with their cultures, vulnerabilities, strengths, and personalities. Religious experiences might include participation in organized religion, joining a faith community, taking a comparative religion course, visiting different houses of worship, and investigating a new religious movement (Williams–Nickelson, 2006). Secular spiritual experiences might include daily prayer, meditation, nature, art, and immersion into sacred texts. All are designed to understand our place in the universe and to connect us to a larger purpose.

The clinician who has found adequate meaning separate and apart from the role of psychotherapist will be better able to enter into this endeavor with enthusiasm and optimism. The practice of psychotherapy is to be pursued to nurture the well-being of the client rather than that of the therapist. The focus remains on the client's needs and concerns, and all efforts are intended to increase meaning in the client's life. The psychotherapist who has found ultimate meaning for her life elsewhere will have no need to compete with clients for time and attention during psychotherapy sessions. It is also easier to set the role of psychotherapist aside at the end of the workday. Hopefully, the practice of psychotherapy remains a meaningful career for the clinician, but it is not the source of greatest meaning in the practitioner's life. It can be surrendered at the end of a session, the end of an extended course of treatment, or at the end of the day. Ultimate meaning lies elsewhere, in the personal life and relationships of the psychotherapist.

Letting Your Life Speak

"Let your life speak" is a time-honored Quaker admonition, usually taken to mean "Let the highest truths and values guide everything you do." It reminds us to live authentically and to embody our values.

Your life speaks by finding your vocations, listening to and accepting your true self, with its limits and potentials. The word *vocation* is rooted in the Latin for "voice." Vocation does not mean a goal that we pursue. It means a calling that we hear. Before we can tell life what we want to do with it, we must listen to our life telling us who we are (Palmer, 2000).

Psychotherapists manifest spirituality by living it daily, in accord with their vocation and values. In his compelling book *Let Your Life Speak*, educator Parker Palmer (2000) describes how anchoring a career in the bedrock of our heartfelt vocational calling is the best way to ensure a long, thriving professional career. We agree and invite you, the reader, to reflect on your earliest memories of the motivations and decisions that led you to become a clinician. What attracted you to this work? Who was most pleased with your choice of work? Who was least pleased and why? What has been your most satisfying moment as a psychotherapist? These memories may serve as precious touchstones that provide meaning, perspective, and renewal throughout the course of a long career. Recall and review them often.

Our discussion hints at a serious concern that merits brief mention, namely, being frustrated by not finding meaning and answers to ultimate concerns in the practice of psychotherapy. It risks pinning too much on the work, the craft, and the therapeutic relationship. Psychotherapy can be pedestrian, even repetitive at times—anything but a transcendent experience. It is not the successful practice of psychotherapy that provides meaning; it is living a deeply personal meaning.

IN CLOSING

We are convinced that the best of who we are, as therapists and indeed as humans, comes from the vitality of the heart. It is the wellspring of the caring and commitment that give meaning to life inside and outside of the consultation room.

This central message, we hope, has been communicated in this chapter in ways that are respectful, ecumenical, and nearly universal. We tried to avoid a particular theocentric slant or subtly imposing our own agendas on very personal, complex topics. Our message is about the self-care imperative of spirituality and mission, not religion per se. We are reminded of Jung's observation that a great deal of religion shields us from religious experience. Spirituality and mission may be manifested through religion, but they are not synonymous with religion.

Pause for a moment to consider spirituality in your life. At the office, is it sufficiently fueling your caring, optimism about human spirit, and commitment to growth? Are you maintaining a high view of work as a high vocation, a calling? Away from the office, are you pursuing sources of personal meaning apart from your work? Are you giving enough time to the relationships of greatest importance in your personal life? Do you participate as a citizen-therapist? Are you addressing the ultimate existential questions of your life? Are you letting your life speak? We beseech you to act worthy of the calling into which you were called, with gentleness, healing, and mission.

The thrust of this chapter is beautifully captured in the words of Laura Brown (2005, p. 956):

I really am a psychotherapist because being one requires me to grow, to consider deeply the existential qualities of life, to find the capacity for joy in the midst of despair. I really am a psychotherapist because the practice of psychotherapy has allowed me to integrate all of me and to continue to pursue *Tikkun olam* every day of my life.

We conclude this chapter with Laura's inspiring words and the renewing benedictions that conclude many religious services: fill our hearts with joy and peace; refresh us as we travel through this wilderness; depart to serve.

SELF-CARE CHECKLIST

✓ Identify and then resonate with your abiding mission in life. What mission do you want written on your tombstone (epitaph)?

✓ Embrace your sense of calling to be a clinician. What are the spiritual antecedents to your career choice?

✓ Cultivate awe and wonder at the human spirit; it will enable you to pull hope from hell.

✓ Invoke and augment your clients' spirituality to enrich their experience of psychotherapy.

✓ Connect to the spiritual sources of your hope and optimism regarding human behavior. If you have lost your enduring sense of caring and concern for others, get help.

✓ Assess periodically your belief in the potential for personality change, a prerequisite for good clinical practice.

✓ Take 10–15 minutes and write a stream of consciousness letter to your God, Nature, Spirit, or a higher power. What did you learn or relearn about your connection to spirituality?

✓ Evaluate the integration of spirituality and personal growth in your own life. How are you doing? What are you doing to promote such a synthesis?

✓ Confront squarely your own yearnings for a sense of transcendence and meaning.

✓ Create a hope-protecting philosophy of life that will help inoculate you from the despair of your clients.

✓ Cherish and practice your *tikkun* (healing and repairing the world).

✓ Pursue the ultimate questions and find meaning in your personal life so that practicing psychotherapy does not become the ultimate meaning for you.

✓ Become a citizen-therapist by merging your vocation with social activism.

✓ Let your life speak—manifest your values and vocation in daily life.

RECOMMENDED READING

Karasu, T. B. (2002). *The art of serenity.* New York: Simon & Schuster.

Kottler, J. A. (2000). *Doing good: Passion and commitment for helping others.* New York: Brunner-Routledge.

Moore, T. (1992). *Care of the soul: A guide for cultivating depth and sacredness in everyday life.* New York: HarperCollins.

Palmer, P. J. (2000). *Let your life speak: Listening for the voice of vocation.* San Francisco: Jossey-Bass.

CHAPTER 12

Fostering Creativity and Growth

We must always change, renew, rejuvenate ourselves;
otherwise we harden.

—JOHANN VON GOETHE

In our roles as psychotherapists, we usefully remind our clients of the centrality of creativity, experimentation, and growth. Witness the number of bromides: "Take risks." "Let's be creative." "Try something different." "Expose yourself to novel situations." "Let's experiment." "Growth involves uncertainty and fear." In our roles as people, by contrast, we tend not to be particularly adventuresome. Like all humans, we are fearful of venturing out on our own into new practice territories, theoretical orientations, and professional activities. Psychotherapists tend to be more conservative in making behavior changes than what they recommend to others. We, the authors, ruefully recognize ourselves in this characterization, by the way.

This inconsistency, or perhaps duplicity, is painfully obvious in the 2005 movie *Prime*. Meryl Streep, the psychotherapist, is encouraging and accepting with her patients but moments later Streep, the mother, is judgmental and intolerant with her children. Our public pronouncements are at odds sometimes with our private behaviors.

What distinguishes the passionately committed psychotherapist from the run-of-the-mill therapist? Adaptiveness and openness to challenges (Dlugos & Friedlander, 2001). Passionately committed therapists score quite high on psychometric measures of openness—seeking new knowl-

197

edge, availing to new experiences, and appreciating ordinary experiences as potentially extraordinary.

Passionate therapists transform obstacles into challenges. A case in point is working with seriously disturbed patients. Passionate therapists move heaven and earth in coordinating first rate care and in providing exceptional service despite the odds. Another case in point is managed care. Most mental health professionals reluctantly participate in managed care systems, a few established colleagues opt out of it altogether and go managed-care free, and a few courageous souls buckle down and creatively work the system. They learn the rules of managed care, develop personal relationships with managed care representatives, use peer support, and capitalize on organizational solutions.

This chapter is devoted to amplified reflections and self-care recommendations on a triad of vital areas: creativity, diversity, and growth. It is imperative to do more than keep our noses above the waterline; we must thrive, not simply survive. As the final chapter in this volume, we also highlight a few points we made earlier and then bid you a fond good-bye.

CREATIVITY

The best psychotherapists are rigorous and logical as well as intuitive and imaginative. Scientific and aesthetic qualities are in high demand in any creative enterprise (Rothenberg, 1988). It is the creative process that often carries us through those wearisome and frustrating hours, days, and years of difficult therapies. Everything comes together for a therapist in the creative process (Kottler, 1999).

Creativity is the state, capacities, and conditions of bringing forth new entities or events that are both new and valuable (Rothenberg, 1988). Examples of creativity in psychotherapy are:

- Appreciating the therapeutic process itself
- Awareness of the paradoxes of treatment (e.g., the patient becomes temporarily dependent on the therapist in order to advance eventual independence)
- Creating of effective metaphors to convey the message
- Experiencing the flash of insight and discovery
- Recognizing irony in the human predicament and psychotherapy itself
- Developing a new and efficacious treatment method

Psychotherapy and self-care are creative processes that emphasize value, innovation, and volition. Both aim for new and valuable ways to understanding, behaving, renewing. Unleash your creativity and pursue self-care activities that light your fire.

Here are two examples from our interviews with master clinicians:

"The main way that I express my creativity is to take a room and remodel it. I find it to be a mental escape and a refreshing break to take a room, strip it to nothing, and then rebuild it. It takes me approximately 1 year to finish a room."

"Novel activities, like go on a mystery night on a cruise ship, have a theme party at the house, travel to unusual places. I might do some unconventional things where I don't have to act professionally."

The important point is to do something, to transform awareness (or insight) into action. In C. S. Lewis's *The Screwtape Letters* (1943), a demon imparts the following advice for capturing souls for Hell to his apprentice:

> The great thing is to prevent his doing anything. As long as he does not convert it into action, it does not matter how much he thinks about his new repentance. . . . Let him do anything but act. The more often he feels without acting, the less he will ever be able to act, and, in the long run, the less he will be able to feel.

So, as you cultivate the skillful attitude for self-care, please translate the creative attitude into behavior and your commitment into corrective activity (lest your soul be lost to the demons!).

The creativity can be actualized in any of the self-care strategies recommended in this book. Be creative in minding your body, nurturing relationships, setting boundaries, sustaining healthy escapes, and so on. And be creative in your professional work, a topic to which we now turn.

DIVERSITY

Creativity is unleashed when we diversify. Here we mean diversity in several distinct senses: diversifying your psychotherapy practice, diversifying your clients, and diversifying your professional activities. The research indicates that such diversification is a protective factor against burnout (Skovholt & Jennings, 2004).

Diversifying your psychotherapy practice essentially means to mix it up. Rearrange your clinical schedule (emphasizing different parts of the day, for example), alter your activities, offer different methods (hypnosis or biofeedback, for example), consider diverse therapy formats (individual, couple, family, group), move the furniture, switch some pictures. We are all at risk of becoming stale.

As much as we enjoy individual therapy, we have made concerted efforts to conduct more couple, family, and group therapy. It requires additional and complementary therapy conceptualizations and skills. It forcibly reminds us of larger systemic and cultural forces. It stretches, expands, and enriches us.

So too does diversifying psychotherapy clients in terms of their characteristics and concerns. Practicing within their clinical competence, of course, practitioners are rewarded with the spice of life by working with patients of a variety of ages, genders, ethnicities, faiths, socioeconomic classes, and diagnostic clusters. Anyone who has seen five straight depressed patients in a row knows exactly of what we speak. Let the next one be anyone but another depressed patient! Far better for the practitioner—and probably for the patient—to intersperse one's schedule with patients presenting with anxiety, relationship, existential, and addictive disorders.

In our own private practices, for instance, we work to diversify our clients. One of us alternates individual psychotherapy sessions with high socioeconomic status mental health professionals with pro bono group therapy with chronic pain patients. One of us mixes patients with addictive disorders and those with mental disorders. Although the patients and diagnoses overlap considerably, the mental health professions and the addiction professions have benignly neglected one another for decades.

In extrapolating from the empirical research on psychotherapists' self-care, we discern a recurring theme: the diversity and synergy of professional activities. The diversity is grounded in performing multiple activities—psychotherapy, assessment, research, writing, teaching, clinical supervision, consultation, and administration. In a study on clinical psychologists (Norcross et al., 2005), we found that half or more of them were routinely involved in all eight of the preceding professional activities.

One of the many benefits of being a psychotherapist is our degrees of freedom. We can write a book, teach others, offer community outreach, consult with agencies and self-help organizations, perform executive coaching, supervise interns, conduct research, lead seminars, evaluate programs, provide divorce mediation, ad infinitum. Multiple benefits accrue from these multiple role functions: our career fulfillment, skill sets, and clinical impact generally increase.

We ourselves have made decisions to diversify in this respect. One of us combines a full-time academic position with editing and a part-time practice. One of us mingles a full-time administrative and clinical position with a private practice. A definite advantage of being a psychotherapist is not being forced to do it exclusively!

Here is how three of our master clinicians add variety to their professional lives by mixing it up:

"If there is a time where a number of my clients don't seem to be doing well, or I feel tired or as though I am not listening well, I may try to re-energize myself by investing time in writing, administrative work, or some reading. After doing some writing or spending some time with my family, I feel like I do have more energy. I am better able to listen to my patients."

"I was involved in 508 television interviews, talk shows, and magazine interviews. I found that it broke up the day to be able to engage in these activities between patients. Along with breaking the monotony of seeing patients all day, it allowed for some further communication and tension reduction between patients and myself."

"Other professional activities, such as teaching and writing, help alleviate the stress of clinical practice. It does so by helping me take one step back from the therapy process. Where I can see the big picture. It eliminates the pressure to do something about an urgent problem. And other professional activities help clarify my thinking."

GROWTH

An essential determinant of professional development is a future orientation, or what has been labeled *possible selves*. Possible selves are aspects of the working self that pertain to what people wish to become and what they are afraid of becoming in the future, that is, hoped-for and feared possible selves. Possible selves are positively associated with seniority and with career satisfaction of psychotherapists (Eshel & Kadouch-Kowalsky, 2003). Research indicates that career satisfaction is contingent on your success in both reducing fears of professional failures (e.g., isolated, impoverished, stale) and enhancing your hope for professional success. Put simply, prevent the worst *and* enhance success in the future.

What is your hoped-for self in the future? We have found imagery work useful here. Take a few private moments to imagine yourself as a psychotherapist in the future, say, 2–5 years from now. What do you want to be doing? What, equally importantly, do you *not* want to be doing? This imagery exercise has led to powerful realizations in our self-care workshops for some participants and modest corrections for some others.

In order to grow, we must constantly make our future rather than only defend our past. Like the two-faced Roman god Janus, we simultaneously look backward and forward. In the Janusian tradition (Rothenberg, 1988), we offer now several prospects for your continued growth not covered elsewhere in this volume.

Continuing Education

In Japanese, *kaizen* means continuous improvement, lifelong learning, and continuing growth. This notion stands in marked contrast to the traditional Western connotation of continuing education as a mandated, typically pedestrian, workshop. We mean continuing education as *kaizen*.

Continued learning is one of the highest-ranked occupational rewards and one of the highest-rated career-sustaining behaviors of psychotherapists (Kramen-Kahn & Hansen, 1998). It might be personal readings, exciting workshops, journal clubs, mentoring, forming a study group, at-home study, or new training opportunities. Whatever it is, it should set your hair on fire—*kaizen*—and actualize your love of lifelong learning.

Jim Bugental (1987, p. 95) reminds us: "An art is not a contest; it's a continual growing. Whenever the artist thinks she's mastered the craft, she's stopped growing and so has stopped being an artist. True art is only found on the edge of what is unknown—a dangerous place to be, an exciting place to work, a continually unsettling place to live subjectively."

Videotape Yourself

Several practitioners (e.g., Lowe, 2005; Mahrer, 2000) periodically videotape their sessions and watch themselves work to maintain their edge and creativity. Most of us did so during our clinical training, with pain and trepidation. It is not nearly as painful to watch later on in one's career, but it is equally educational. We see things that we missed in our clients. It helps us remain alert and focused in following sessions. Remember: even world-class athletes continue to look at videos of themselves in action to stay on top of their game (Lowe, 2005).

Professional Organizations

A recurrent comment from master clinicians is that their self-care is spurred by active engagement with professional organizations. In part, this occurs because it provides diversity in weekly activities; in part, because of the nourishing relationships; and in part, because we join like-minded people in forwarding and shaping the mission of our art/science. We encourage you to become active in the governance of local, state, national, or international organizations.

Interdisciplinary Inquiry

Recent years have brought unprecedented opportunities for psychotherapists to participate in fascinating interdisciplinary investigations of fundamental human questions. The study of attachment, consciousness, autonomy, and creativity itself is informed by our clinical findings and our research expertise. The urgent press for sociopsychological intervention in human suffering—terrorism, poverty, fanaticism, racism—cries out for mental health contributions, locally and nationally. We urge you to invest in interdisciplinary movements to investigate and help remedy the cries of the world.

JUST A FEW WORDS BEFORE WE GO

In this, our final chapter, we would like to come full circle by returning briefly to our overarching goals for the book. You may recall that, in the Preface, we characterized *Leaving It at the Office* as a curious mix of a "how-to," "you should," and "chill-out" manual. We hope that the practical, "how-to" self-care orientation came through clearly in our text, examples, research findings, and Self-Care Checklists. Without sounding judgmental, the "you should" emphasis tried to remind you of the compelling ethics, research, and experience that you should replenish yourself. Doing so enhances you as a person and as a professional. The "chill-out" injunction is the collegial reminder that universal prescriptions for self-care do not, and cannot, fit us all. Different strokes for different folks. We all need something a little different; as Lord Byron put it, we are all differently organized.

Our ardent hope is that our book gently and collegially reminds you that our lives are works in progress and that you can practice self-care wholeheartedly as a skillful attitude. Not every psychotherapist can be expected to master or profit from all self-care possibilities.

Nor, more broadly, can any psychotherapist's life be perfect. When the personal life is necessarily imperfect, therapists are prone to think and feel that something is wrong and inclined to fault themselves. This tendency is often associated with painful and unwarranted inferences that they are lousy therapists ("because I don't have my own life together"), imposters ("I am only playing at the role of an expert, but if my clients only knew the truth!"), or suffer from the Moses complex ("I can lead others to the promised land of health, but cannot enter it myself"; Mahoney, 2003).

Please be gentle with yourself. We psychotherapists bear a heavy burden of expectations that we must be unusually happy, wise, and empathic for others in order to feel we are "true" professionals.

We, the authors, struggle with our own self-care, but it is improving bit by bit. Over the years, John has become more selective with the clients he accepts, declines most offers to give workshops, maintains his part-time practice at one long day per week, accepts only high-reward projects, says "no" more often, insists on 8 hours of sleep (10:00 P.M. bedtime), and exercises three times a week (well, most weeks, anyway). But he still needs to work less, improve his diet, and communicate more meaningfully with his spouse and kids. In recent years, Jim has come to appreciate that maintaining close relationships with his spouse and children is more satisfying and meaningful than ambitiously pursuing career goals. He repeatedly evaluates and reorganizes his work priorities to match the evolving needs of his family. And we (John and Jim) are both tempering our high-achievement dictates that our self-care ought to be perfect.

AVE ATQUE VALE

Reading the literature, surveying our colleagues, conducting workshops, and writing this book have aided immeasurably in the practice of our own self-care. Research on self-care—classified as "mesearch" in academia—helped to center and balance us. Thank you for your participation and companionship in joining us on the journey.

Thus, we bid you a fond *ave atque vale*—hail and farewell. We hope that a few of our words, examples, and self-care methods go with you. Keep the self-care faith, and spread it when you can.

IN CLOSING

Self-care is not a list one checks off in the morning and is done with; no, it is a skillful attitude and lifelong commitment.

We should expect a lifetime of struggling for awareness and pursuing growth. Ever repeated confrontations with our personal and public selves are necessary for fulfillment. We cannot, like the biblical Isaac, spend just one night wrestling with an angel to win his blessing (Guggenbuhl-Craig, 1971). The struggle will last a lifetime.

The gift of self-renewal is the process of creativity and growth. In the end, we can do more than survive—we can thrive. Ram Dass reminds us that the purpose of the dance is not to finish. The purpose of the dance is to dance! May we all dance 'til we drop.

SELF-CARE CHECKLIST

✓ Strive for adaptiveness and openness to challenges—the defining characteristics of passionately committed psychotherapists.

✓ Upgrade your creativity through innovative treatments, valuable metaphors, therapeutic irony, and novel methods.

✓ Diversify, diversify, diversify. Involvement in diverse professional activities balances your workload and expresses the full array of your skills.

✓ Mix up your therapy days: individual, couple, group, and family formats; younger and older patients; talk therapy and action therapy. What else can you do to increase variety and novelty in your schedule?

✓ Imagine periodically your future possible selves as a psychotherapist and then set sail in that direction.

✓ Embrace continuing education as *kaizen*—continuous improvement and lifelong learning.

✓ Attend clinical conferences, read literature, and form study groups to access the life springs of a committed professional. Do you feel you are just getting continuing education hours or refining and expanding your skills?

✓ Engage actively with professional organizations to shape our collective mission and to keep yourself involved.

✓ Create your own personal mission statement to sharpen your focus and prioritize your activities.

✓ Convert the skillful attitude of self-care into concrete behavior—lest your soul be lost to the demons!

✓ Invest in interdisciplinary movements to investigate and help remedy cries of distress in the world.

✓ Be gentle with yourself—shed the heavy burden of expectations about personal perfection that psychotherapists carry.

✓ Expect a lifetime of struggle for awareness and growth; self-renewal is a long-term process of creativity and growth.

RECOMMENDED READING

Koocher, G. P., Norcross, J. C., & Hill, S. S. (Eds.). (2005). *Psychologists' desk reference* (2nd ed.). New York: Oxford University Press.

Kottler, J. A. (1999). *The therapist's workbook: Self-assessment, self-care, and self-improvement exercises for mental health professionals*. San Francisco: Jossey-Bass.

Kottler, J. A. (2003). *On being a therapist* (3rd ed.). San Francisco: Jossey-Bass.

Orlinsky, D. E., & Rønnestad, M. H. (2005). *How psychotherapists develop: A study of therapeutic work and professional growth*. Washington, DC: American Psychological Association.

Rothenberg, A. (1988). *The creative process of psychotherapy*. New York: Norton.

References

Abend, S. (1986). Countertransference, empathy, and the analytic ideal. *Psychoanalytic Quarterly, 55,* 563–575.

American Counseling Association. (2005). *ACA code of ethics.* Alexandria, VA: Author.

American Psychological Association. (2002). Ethical principles of psychologists and code of conduct. *American Psychologist, 57,* 1060–1073.

American Psychological Association. (2006). *Advancing colleague assistance in professional psychology.* Washington, DC: Author.

Ashway, J. A. (1984). A therapist's pregnancy: An opportunity for conflict resolution and growth in the treatment of children. *Clinical Social Work Journal, 121,* 3–17.

Baker, E. K. (2003). *Caring for ourselves: A therapist's guide to personal and professional well-being.* Washington, DC: American Psychological Association.

Balint, M. (1957). *The doctor, his patient and the illness.* New York: International University Press.

Balsam, A., & Balsam, R. (1974). The pregnant therapist. In A. Balsam & R. Balsam (Eds.), *On becoming a psychotherapist* (pp. 265–288). Boston: Little, Brown.

Barbanelli, L. H. (1986). The selfless caretaker. *Psychotherapy Patient, 2,* 105–109.

Barnett, J. E., & Hillard, D. (2001). Psychologist distress and impairment: The availability, nature, and use of colleague assistance programs for psychologists. *Professional Psychology: Research and Practice, 32,* 205–210.

Barnett, J. E., Johnston, L. C., & Hillard, D. (2006). Psychotherapist wellness as an ethical imperative. In L. VandeCreek & J. B. Allen (Eds.), *Innovations in clinical practice: Focus on health and wellness* (pp. 257–271). Sarasota, FL: Professional Resources Press.

Barron, J. W. (1999). *Humor and psyche: Psychoanalytic perspectives.* Hillsdale, NJ: Analytic Press.

207

Barrow, J. C., English, T., & Pinkerton, R. S. (1987). Physical fitness training: Beneficial for professional psychologists? *Professional Psychology: Research and Practice, 18*, 66–70.

Baumeister, R. F. (1992). *Escaping the self: Alcoholism, spirituality, masochism, and other flights from the burden of selfhood*. New York: Basic Books.

Beck, A. T., Rush, J. A., Shaw, B. F., & Emery, G. (1979). *Cognitive therapy of depression*. New York: Guilford Press.

Beck, J. S. (1997, August). *Cognitive therapy methods for self-care*. Paper presented at the 105th annual convention of the American Psychological Association, Chicago.

Beck, J. S., & Butler, A. C. (2005). Treating psychotherapists with cognitive therapy. In J. D. Geller, J. C. Norcross, & D. E. Orlinsky (Eds.), *The psychotherapist's own psychotherapy*. New York: Oxford University Press.

Bellow, S. (1964). *Herzog*. New York: Viking.

Bergin, A. E., & Jensen, J. P. (1990). Religiosity of psychotherapists: A national survey. *Psychotherapy, 27*, 3–7.

Berkowitz, M. (1987) Therapist survival: Maximizing generativity and minimizing burnout. *Psychotherapy in Private Practice, 5*, 85–89.

Betcher, R. W., & Zinberg, N. E. (1988). Supervision and privacy in psychotherapy training. *American Journal of Psychiatry, 145*, 796–803.

Bienen, M. (1990). The pregnant therapist: Countertransference dilemmas and willingness to explore transference material. *Psychotherapy, 27*, 607–612.

Bloch, S., Browning, S., & McGrath, G. (1983). Humour in group psychotherapy. *British Journal of Medical Psychotherapy, 56*, 89–97.

Boice, R., & Myers, P. E. (1987). Which setting is healthier and happier, academe or private practice? *Professional Psychology: Research and Practice, 18*, 526–529.

Bongar, B. (1991). *The suicidal patient: Clinical and legal standards of care*. Washington DC: American Psychological Association.

Bootzin, R. R. (2005). Stimulus control instructions for the treatment of insomnia. In G. P. Koocher, J. C. Norcross, & S. S. Hill (Eds.), *Psychologists' desk reference* (2nd ed.). New York: Oxford University Press.

Borys, D. S., & Pope, K. S. (1989). Dual relationships between therapist and client. *Professional Psychology: Research and Practice, 20*, 283–293.

Bowen, M. (1972). On the differentiation of self. In J. Framo (Ed.), *Family interaction: A dialogue between family researchers and family therapists*. New York: Springer.

Boylin, W. M., & Briggie, C. R. (1987).The healthy therapist: The contribution of the symbolic-experiential family therapy. *Family Therapy, 14*, 247–256.

Brady, J. L., Guy, J. D., Poelstra, P. L., & Brokaw, B. F. (1999). Vicarious traumatization, spirituality, and the treatment of sexual abuse survivors: A national survey of women psychotherapists. *Professional Psychology: Research and Practice, 30*, 386–393.

Brady, J. L., Guy, J. D., Poelstra, P. L., & Brown, C. K. (1996). Difficult goodbyes: A national survey of therapists' hindrances to successful terminations. *Psychotherapy in Private Practice, 14*, 65–76.

Brady, J. L., Healy, F. C., Norcross, J. C., & Guy, J. D. (1995). Stress in counsellors: An integrative research review. In W. Dryden (Ed.), *The stresses of counselling in action*. London: Sage.

Brady, J. L., Norcross, J. C., & Guy, J. D. (1995). Managing your own distress: Lessons from psychotherapists healing themselves. In L. VandeCreek, S. Knapp, & T. L. Jackson (Eds.), *Innovations in clinical practice* (pp. 293–306). Sarasota, FL: Professional Resource Press.

Bromfield, R. (1996). Being true to thyself, an ethical obligation. *APA Monitor on Psychology, 27*(10), 14.

Brooks, G. R. (1990). The inexpressive male and vulnerability to therapist–patient sexual exploitation. *Psychotherapy, 27*, 344–349.

Brown, H. N. (1987). Patient suicide during residency training: Incidence, implications, and program response. *Journal of Psychiatric Education, 11*, 201–206.

Brown, L. S. (2005). Don't be a sheep: How this eldest daughter became a feminist therapist. *Journal of Clinical Psychology: In Session, 61*, 949–956.

Browne, J. (1974). Fountain of sorrow. Song lyrics on Asylum Records LP *Late for the sky.*

Buchholz, E. S. (1997). *The call of solitude: Alonetime in a world of attachment.* New York: Simon & Schuster.

Buckley, P., Karasu, T. B., & Charles, E. (1981). Psychotherapists view their personal therapy. *Psychotherapy, 18*, 299–305.

Bugental, J. F. T. (1964). The person who is the psychotherapist. *Journal of Consulting Psychology, 28*, 272–277.

Bugental, J. F. T. (1978). *Psychotherapy and process.* Reading, MA: Addison-Wesley.

Bugental, J. F. T. (1987). *The art of the psychotherapist.* New York: Norton.

Burton, A. (1969). To seek and encounter critical people. *Voices, 5*, 26–28.

Burton, A. (Ed.). (1972). *Twelve therapists: How they live and actualize themselves.* San Francisco: Jossey-Bass.

Cady, S. H., & Jones, G. E. (1997). Massage therapy as a workplace intervention for reduction of stress. *Perceptual and Motor Skills, 84*, 157–158.

Cann, A., Holt, K., & Calhoun, L. G. (1999). The roles of humor and sense of humor in responses to stressors. *International Journal of Humor Research, 12*, 177–193.

Canter, M. B. (1997). Physician heal thyself? Yes, but . . . *Psychotherapy in Private Practice, 16*, 11–18.

Carroll, L., Gilroy, P. J., & Murra, J. (1999). The moral imperative: Self-care for women psychotherapists. *Women and Therapy, 22*, 133–143.

Chemtob, C. M., Bauer, G. B., Hamada, R. S., Pelowski, S. R., & Muraoka, M. Y. (1989). Patient suicide: Occupational hazard for psychologists and psychiatrists. *Professional Psychology: Research and Practice, 20*, 294–300.

Chessick, R. D. (1990). Self-analysis: A fool for a patient? *Psychoanalytic Review, 40*, 311–340.

Chodron, P. (1994). *Start where you are: A guide to compassionate living.* Boston: Shambala.

Clark, M. M. (1986). Personal therapy: A review of empirical research. *Professional Psychology: Research and Practice, 17*, 541–543.

Clifton, D., Doan, R., & Mitchell, D. (1990). The reauthoring of therapist's stories: Taking doses of our own medicine. *Journal of Strategic and Systemic Therapies, 9*, 61–66.

Cogan, T. (1977). A study of friendship among psychotherapists (Doctoral dissertation, Illinois Institute of Technology). *Dissertation Abstracts International, 78,* 859.

Corey, M. S., & Corey, G. (1989). *Becoming a helper.* Pacific Grove, CA: Brooks/Cole.

Coster, J. S., & Schwebel, M. (1997). Well-functioning in professional psychologists. *Professional Psychology: Research and Practice, 28,* 5–13.

Covey, S. R. (1989). *The 7 habits of highly effective people.* New York: Simon & Schuster.

Crits-Christoph, P., Baranackie, K., Kurcias, J. S., Beck, A. T., Carroll, K., Perry, K., et al. (1991). Meta-analysis of therapist effects in psychotherapy outcome studies. *Psychotherapy Research, 2,* 81–91.

Cummings, N. A. (1986). The dismantling of our health system: Strategies for the survival of psychological practice. *American Psychologist, 41,* 426–431.

Cummings, N. A. (1988). Emergence of the mental health complex: Adaptive and maladaptive responses. *Professional Psychology: Research and Practice, 19,* 308–315.

Dement, W. C., & Vaughan, C. (2000). *The promise of sleep.* New York: Dell.

Deutsch, C. J. (1984). Self-reported sources of stress among psychotherapists. *Professional Psychology: Research and Practice, 15,* 833–845.

Deutsch, C. J. (1985). A survey of therapists' personal problems and treatment. *Professional Psychology: Research and Practice, 16,* 305–315.

Dewald, P. A. (1982). Serious illness in the analyst: Transference, countertransference, and reality responses. *Journal of the American Psychoanalytic Association, 30,* 347–363.

Dickinson, E. (1890/2001). *Poems.* Retrieved on February 26, 2007, from *http://www.gutenberg.org/dirs/etext01/1mlyd10.txt.*

DiMatteo, M. R. (2006). Enhancing adherence. In G. P. Koocher, J. C. Norcross, & S. S. Hill (Eds.), *Psychologists' desk reference.* New York: Oxford University Press.

Dlugos, R. F., & Friedlander, M. L. (2001). Passionately committed psychotherapists: A qualitative study of their experiences. *Professional Psychology: Research and Practice, 32,* 298–304.

Dorken, H. (1990). Malpractice claims experience of psychologists: Policy issues, cost comparisons with psychiatrists, and prescription privilege applications. *Professional Psychology: Research and Practice, 21,* 150–152.

Doyle, B. B. (1987). The impaired psychiatrist. *Psychiatric Annals, 17,* 760–763.

Dryden, W. (Ed.). (1995). *The stresses of counselling in action.* London: Sage.

Dryden, W., & Spurling, L. (Eds.). (1989). *On becoming a psychotherapist.* London: Routledge.

Dumont, M. (1992). Privatization of mental health services: The invisible hand at our throats. *American Journal of Orthopsychiatry, 62,* 328–329.

Edelwich, J., & Brodsky, A. (1980). *Burn-out.* New York: Human Sciences Press.

Edelwich, J., & Brodsky, A. (1991). *Sexual dilemmas for the helping professional.* New York: Brunner/Mazel.

Ekstein, R., & Wallerstein, R. S. (1972). *The teaching and learning of psychotherapy* (2nd ed.). New York: International University Press.

Eliot, T. S. (1992). Four quarters: Burnt Norton. In *The complete poems and plays, 1909–1950.* New York: Harcourt Brace.

Elliot, D. M., & Guy, J. D. (1993). Mental health professionals versus non-mental health professionals: Childhood trauma and adult functioning. *Professional Psychology: Research and Practice, 24,* 83–90.

Elliott, R., & James, E. (1989). Varieties of client experience in psychotherapy: An analysis of the literature. *Clinical Psychology Review, 9,* 443–467.

Ellis, A. (1984). How to deal with your most difficult client–you. *Psychotherapy in Private Practice, 2,* 25–35.

Ellis, A. (1987). The impossibility of achieving consistently good mental health. *American Psychologist, 42,* 364–375.

Ellis, A. (1995, August). *How I manage to be a "rational" rational emotive behavior therapist.* Paper presented at the 103rd annual convention of the American Psychological Association, New York.

Ellis, T. E., & Dickey, T. O. (1998). Procedures surrounding the suicide of a trainee's patient: A national survey of psychology internship and psychiatry residency programs. *Professional Psychology: Research and Practice, 29,* 492–497.

Epstein, R. S. (1994). *Keeping boundaries: Maintaining safety and integrity in the psychotherapeutic process.* Washington, DC: American Psychiatric Press.

Eshel, Y., & Kadouch-Kowalsky, J. (2003). Professional possible selves, anxiety, and seniority as determinants of professional satisfaction of psychotherapists. *Psychotherapy Research, 13,* 429–442.

Farber, B. A. (1983a). Dysfunctional aspects of the therapeutic role. In B. A. Farber (Ed.), *Stress and burnout in the human service profession* (pp. 97–118). New York: Pergamon.

Farber, B. A. (1983b). The effects of psychotherapeutic practice upon psychotherapists. *Psychotherapy, 20,* 174–182.

Farber, B. A. (1983c). Psychotherapists' perceptions of stressful patient behavior. *Professional Psychology: Research and Practice, 14,* 697–705.

Farber, B. A. (1990). Burnout in psychotherapists: Incidence, types, and trends. *Psychotherapy in Private Practice, 8,* 35–44.

Farber, B. A. (1998, August). *Tailoring treatment strategies for different types of burnout.* Paper presented at the annual meeting of the American Psychological Association, San Francisco, CA.

Farber, B. A., & Heifetz, L. J. (1981). The satisfactions and stresses of psychotherapeutic work: A factor analytic study. *Professional Psychology: Research and Practice, 12,* 621–630.

Farber, B. A., & Heifetz, L. J. (1982). The process and dimensions of burnout in psychotherapists. *Professional Psychology, 13,* 293–301.

Farber, B. A., & Norcross, J. C. (Eds.). (2005). Why I (really) became a psychotherapist. *Journal of Clinical Psychology: In Session, 61*(8).

Farber, N. K. (2000). Trainees' Attitudes Toward Seeking Psychotherapy Scale: Development and validation of a research instrument. *Psychotherapy, 37,* 341–353.

Fenster, S., Phillips, S., & Rappoport, E. (1986). *The therapist's pregnancy: Intrusion in the analytic space.* Hillsdale, NJ: Analytic Press.

Fiedler, F. E. (1950a). Comparison of therapeutic relationships in psychoanalytic, non-directive, and Adlerian therapy. *Journal of Consulting Psychology, 14,* 436–445.

Fiedler, F. E. (1950b). The concept of the ideal therapeutic relationship. *Journal of Consulting Psychology, 14,* 239–245.

Field, T. M. (1998). Massage therapy effects. *American Psychologist, 53,* 1270–1281.

Fields, R. (1984). *Chop wood, carry water.* New York: Penguin.

Figley, C. R. (1995). Compassion fatigue as secondary traumatic stress disorder: An overview. In C. R. Figley (Ed.), *Compassion fatigue* (pp. 1–20). New York: Brunner/Mazel.

Firth-Cozens, J. (1992). The role of early family experiences in the perception of organizational stress: Fusing clinical and organizational perspectives. *Journal of Occupational and Organizational Psychology, 65,* 61–75.

Forrest, L., Elman, N., Gizara, S., & Vacha-Haase, T. (1999). Trainee impairment: A review of identification, remediation, dismissal, and legal issues. *The Counseling Psychologist, 27,* 712–721.

Fox, D. (1998). There's no one to heal in the desert. *Psychotherapy Networker, 22*(3), 104–105.

Freeman, W. (1968). *The psychiatrist: Personalities and patterns.* New York: Grune & Stratton.

Fremont, S. K., & Anderson, W. (1988). Investigation of factors involved in therapists' annoyance with clients. *Professional Psychology: Research and Practice, 19,* 330–335.

Freud, S. (1933). Fragment of an analysis of a case of hysteria. In J. Strachey (Ed. and Trans.), *The standard edition of the complete psychological works of Sigmund Freud* (Vol. VII). London: Hogarth Press. (Original work published 1905)

Freud, S. (1957). The future prospects of psychoanalytic therapy. In J. Strachey (Ed. and Trans.), *The standard edition of the complete psychological works of Sigmund Freud* (Vol. X). London: Hogarth Press. (Original work published 1910)

Freud, S. (1964). Recommendations to physicians practicing psychoanalysis. In J. Strachey (Ed. and Trans.), *The standard edition of the complete psychological works of Sigmund Freud* (Vol. XII). London: Hogarth Press. (Original work published 1912)

Freud, S. (1964). Analysis terminable and interminable. In J. Strachey (Ed. and Trans.), *The standard edition of the complete psychological works of Sigmund Freud* (Vol. XXIII). London: Hogarth Press. (Original work published 1937)

Freudenberger, H. J. (1975). The staff burn-out syndrome in alternative institutions. *Psychotherapy: Theory, Research, and Practice, 12,* 73–82.

Freudenberger, H. J. (1983). Hazards of psychotherapeutic practice. *Psychotherapy in Private Practice, 1,* 83–89.

Freudenberger, H. J. (1990a). Therapists as men and men as therapists. *Psychotherapy, 27,* 340–343.

Freudenberger, H. J. (1990b). Hazards of psychotherapeutic practice. *Psychotherapy in Private Practice, 8,* 31–34.

Freudenberger, H. J., & Kurtz, T. (1990). Risks and rewards of independent practice. In E. A. Margenau (Ed.), *The encyclopedic handbook of private practice* (pp. 461–472). New York: Gardner.

Freudenberger, H. J., & Richelson, G. (1980). *Burn out: How to beat the high cost of success.* New York: Bantam.

Freudenberger, H. J., & Robbins, A. (1979). The hazards of being a psychoanalyst. *Psychoanalytic Review, 66,* 275–295.

Frisina, P. G., Borod, J. C., & Lepore, S. J. (2004). A meta-analysis of the effects of written emotional disclosure on the health outcomes of clinical populations. *Journal of Nervous and Mental Disease, 192,* 629–634.

Gadzella, B. M., Ginther, D. W., Tomcala, M., & Bryant, G. W. (1991). Educators' appraisal of their stressors and coping strategies. *Psychological Reports, 68,* 995–998.

Galanter, M., Larson, D., & Rubenstone, E. (1991). Christian psychiatry: The impact of evangelical belief on clinical practice. *American Journal of Psychiatry, 148,* 90–95.

Gamble, S. J., Pearlman, L. A., Lucca, A. M., & Allen, G. J. (1994, October). *Differential therapist stressors in psychotherapy with trauma vs. non-trauma clients.* Paper presented at the New England Psychological Association conference, Hamden, CT.

Gardiner, M. (1971). *The wolf-man by the wolf-man.* New York: Basic Books.

Gartrell, N. (2004, January 4). A doctor's toxic shock. *New York Times Magazine,* p. 58.

Geller, J. D., Norcross, J. C., & Orlinsky, D. E. (Eds.). (2005). *The psychotherapist's own psychotherapy: Patient and clinician perspectives.* New York: Oxford University Press.

Gelso, C. J., & Hayes, J. H. (2002). The management of countertransference. In J. C. Norcross (Ed.), *Psychotherapy relationships that work.* New York: Oxford University Press.

Gentile, S., Asamne, J., Harmell, P., & Weathers, R. (2002). The stalking of psychologists by their clients. *Professional Psychology: Research and Practice, 33,* 490–494.

Gershefski, J. J., Arnkoff, D. B., Glass, C. R., & Elkin, I. (1996). Clients' perceptions of their treatment for depression: I. Helpful aspects. *Psychotherapy Research, 6,* 245–259.

Gilligan, C. (1982). *In a different voice: Psychological theory and women's development.* Cambridge, MA: Harvard University Press.

Gladding, S. T. (1991). Counselor self-abuse. *Journal of Mental Health Counseling, 13,* 414–419.

Goldberg, C. (1986). *On being a psychotherapist.* New York: Gardner.

Goldberg, C. (1992). *The seasoned psychotherapist–triumph over adversity.* New York: Norton.

Goldberg, C. (1993). The unexplored in self-analysis. *Psychotherapy, 30,* 159–161.

Golden, V., & Farber, B. A. (1998). Therapists as parents: Is it good for the children? *Professional Psychology: Research and Practice, 29,* 135–139.

Goldfried, M. R. (Ed.). (2001). *How therapists change.* Washington, DC: American Psychological Association.

Goldin, E., & Bordin, T. (1999). The use of humor in counseling: The laughing cure. *Journal of Counseling and Development, 77,* 405–410.

Goldstein, J. H. (1982). A laugh a day: Can mirth keep disease at bay? *The Sciences, 22,* 21–25.

Gottfredson, G. D. (1987). Employment setting, specialization, and patterns of accomplishment among psychologists. *Professional Psychology: Research and Practice, 18,* 452–460.

Graham, S. R. (1995). "A modest proposal." *The Psychotherapy Bulletin, 30,* 4–5.

Gram, A. M. (1992). Peer relationships among clinicians as an alternative to mentor–protégée relationships in hospital settings. *Professional Psychology: Research and Practice, 23,* 416–417.

Greenberg, R. P., & Staller, J. S. (1981). Personal therapy for therapists. *American Journal of Psychiatry, 138,* 1467–1471.

Greenburg, S. L., Lewis, G. J., & Johnson, M. (1985). Peer consultation groups for private practitioners. *Professional Psychology: Research and Practice, 16,* 437–446.

Greenfeld, D. (1985). Stresses of the psychotherapeutic role. *Hillside Journal of Clinical Psychiatry, 7,* 165–182.

Gregory, B. A., & Gilbert, L. A. (1992). The relationship between dependency behavior in female clients and psychologists' perceptions of seductiveness. *Professional Psychology: Research and Practice, 23,* 390–396.

Grodzki, L. (2003). Our businesses, our selves. *Psychotherapy Networker, 27,* 50–59.

Grosch, W. N., & Olsen, D. C. (1994). *When helping starts to hurt: A new look at burnout among psychotherapists.* New York: Norton.

Grunebaum, H. (1983). A study of therapists' choice of a therapist. *American Journal of Psychiatry, 140,* 1336–1339.

Grusky, Z. (1987). The practice of psychotherapy: A search for principles in an ambiguous art. *Psychotherapy, 24,* 1–5.

Guggenbuhl-Craig, A. (1971). *Power in the helping relationships.* Dallas: Spring.

Guntrip, H. (1971). *Psychoanalytic theory, therapy, and the self.* New York: Basic Books.

Gutheil, T. G. (1989). Borderline personality disorder, boundary violations, and patient–therapist sex. *American Journal of Psychiatry, 146,* 597–602.

Guy, J. D. (1987). *The personal life of the psychotherapist.* New York: Wiley.

Guy, J. D. (2000). Holding the holding environment together: Self-psychology and psychotherapist care. *Professional Psychology: Research and Practice, 31,* 351–352.

Guy, J. D., & Brown, C. K. (1992). How to benefit emotionally from private practice. *Psychotherapy in Private Practice, 10,* 27–39.

Guy, J. D., & Brown, C. K. (1993). Necessary losses, legitimate mourning? Psychotherapists' experience of loss during a planned termination. *Voices, 29,* 44–49.

Guy, J. D., Brown, C. K., & Poelstra, P. L. (1990a). Psychotherapist as victim: A discussion of patient violence. *The California Psychologist, 22,* 20–22.

Guy, J. D., Brown, C. K., & Poelstra, P. L. (1990b). Who gets attacked? A national survey of patient violence directed at psychologists in clinical practice. *Professional Psychology: Research and Practice, 21,* 493–495.

Guy, J. D., Brown, C. K., & Poelstra, P. L. (1991). Living with the aftermath: A national survey of the consequences of patient violence directed at psychotherapists. *Psychotherapy in Private Practice, 9,* 35–39.

Guy, J. D., Brown, C. K., & Poelstra, P. L. (1992). Safety concerns and protective measures used by psychotherapists. *Professional Psychology: Research and Practice, 23,* 421–423.

Guy, J. D., French, R. J, Poelstra, P. L., & Brown, C. K. (1993). Therapeutic terminations: How therapists say good-bye. *Psychotherapy in Private Practice, 12,* 73–82.

Guy, J. D., Freudenberger, H., Farber, B., & Norcross, J. C. (1990). Hazards of the psychotherapeutic profession. *Psychotherapy in Private Practice, 8*, 27–61.

Guy, J. D., Guy, M. P., & Liaboe, G. P. (1986). First pregnancy: Therapeutic issues for both female and male psychotherapists. *Psychotherapy, 23*, 297–302.

Guy, J. D., & Liaboe, G. P. (1986). The impact of conducting psychotherapy on psychotherapists' interpersonal functioning. *Professional Psychology: Research and Practice, 17*, 111–114.

Guy, J. D., Poelstra, P. L., & Stark, M. J. (1988). Personal therapy for psychotherapists before and after entering professional practice: A national survey of factors related to its utilization. *Professional Psychology: Research and Practice, 19*, 474–476.

Guy, J. D., Poelstra, P. L., & Stark, M. J. (1989). Personal distress and therapeutic effectiveness: National survey of psychologists practicing psychotherapy. *Professional Psychology: Research and Practice, 20*, 48–50.

Guy, J. D., & Souder, J. K. (1986a). Impact of therapists' illness or accident on psychotherapeutic practice: Review and discussion. *Professional Psychology: Research and Practice, 17*, 509–513.

Guy, J. D., & Souder, J. K. (1986b). The aging psychotherapist. *The Independent Practitioner, 6*, 40–65.

Guy, J. D., Souder, J. K., Baker, R., & Guy, M. P. (1987). Husband and wife psychotherapists: Unique issues and concerns. *Voices, 23*, 56–69.

Guy, J. D., Stark, M. J., Poelstra, P. L., & Souder, J. K. (1987). Psychotherapist retirement and age-related impairment: A national survey and discussion of the issues. *Psychotherapy, 24*, 814–818.

Guy, J. D., Tamura, L. J., & Poelstra, P. L. (1989). All in the family: Multiple therapists per household. *Psychotherapy in Private Practice, 7*, 103–113.

Hage, S. M. (2006). A closer look at the role of spirituality in psychology training programs. *Professional Psychology: Research and Practice, 37*, 303–310.

Haller, R. M., & Deluty, R. H. (1988). Assaults on staff by psychiatric in-patients: A critical review. *British Journal of Psychiatry, 152*, 174–179.

Harlow, H. F. (1958). The nature of love. *American Psychologist, 13*, 573–685.

Harris, E. A., & Bennett, B. E. (2005). Sample psychotherapist–patient contract. In G. P. Koocher, J. C. Norcross, & S. S. Hill (Eds.), *Psychologists' desk reference* (2nd ed.). New York: Oxford University Press.

Hays, K. F. (1995). Psychotherapy and exercise behavior change. *Psychotherapy Bulletin, 30*(3), 29–35.

Hellman, I. D., & Morrison, T. L. (1987). Practice setting and type of caseload as factors in psychotherapist stress. *Psychotherapy, 24*, 427–433.

Hellman, I. D., Morrison, T. L., & Abramowitz, S. I. (1986). The stresses of psychotherapeutic work: A replication and extension. *Journal of Clinical Psychology, 42*, 197–204.

Hellman, I. D., Morrison, T. L., & Abramowitz, S. I. (1987). Therapist flexibility/rigidity and work stress. *Professional Psychology: Research and Practice, 18*, 21–27.

Hendin, H., Haas, A. P., Maltsberger, J. T., Szanton, K., et al. (2004). Factors contributing to therapists' distress after the suicide of a patient. *American Journal of Psychiatry, 161*, 1442–1446.

Henry, W. E., Sims, J. H., & Spray, S. L. (1971). *The fifth profession: Becoming a psychotherapist.* San Francisco: Jossey-Bass.

Henry, W. E., Sims, J. H., & Spray, S. L. (1973). *Public and private lives of psychotherapists.* San Francisco: Jossey-Bass.

Henry, W. P. (1998). Science, politics, and the politics of science: The use and misuse of empirically validated treatment research. *Psychotherapy Research, 8,* 126–140.

Heuser, J. E. (1980). The role of humor and folklore theme in psychotherapy. *American Journal of Psychotherapy, 137,* 1546–1549.

Hoeksema, J. H., Guy, J. D., Brown, C. K., & Brady, J. L. (1993). The relationship between psychotherapist burnout and satisfaction with leisure activities. *Psychotherapy in Private Practice, 12,* 51–59.

Hoff, S., & Buchholz, E. S. (1996). School psychologist know thyself: Creativity and alonetime for adaptive professional coping. *Psychology in the Schools, 33,* 309–317.

Holt, R., & Lubosky, L. (1958). *Personality patterns of psychiatrists.* New York: Basic Books.

Holzman, L. A., Searight, H. R., & Hughes, H. M. (1996). Clinical psychology graduate students and personal psychotherapy: Results of an exploratory survey. *Professional Psychology: Research and Practice, 27,* 98–101.

House, R. (1995). The stress of working in a general practice setting. In W. Dryden & V. Varma (Eds.), *Stresses of counseling in action.* London: Sage.

Institute of Medicine. (2006). Retrieved on July 25, 2006, from *www.iom.edu.*

James, W. (1910). *The principles of psychology.* New York: Dover.

Jamison, K. R. (1997). *An unquiet mind.* New York: Random House.

Janis, T. L. (1958). *Psychological stress.* New York: Wiley.

Janzen, W. B., & Myers, D. V. (1981). Assertion for therapists: A professional bill of rights. *Psychotherapy, 18,* 291–298.

Japenga, A. (1989, April 9). Analyzing psychiatrists' kids: Sons and daughters sound off. *Los Angeles Times,* 1, 14.

Johnston, S. H., & Farber, B. A. (1996). The maintenance of boundaries in psychotherapeutic practice. *Psychotherapy, 33,* 391–402.

Jones, E. (1955). *The life and work of Sigmund Freud: Years of maturity* (Vol. 2). New York: Basic Books.

Jones, S. L. (1994). A constructive relationship for religion with the science and profession of psychology. *American Psychologist, 49,* 184–199.

Kahn, W. L., & Harkavy-Friedman, J. M. (1997). Change in the therapist: The role of patient-induced inspiration. *American Journal of Psychotherapy, 51,* 403–414.

Kaslow, F. W., & Schulman, N. (1987). How to be sane and happy as a family therapist. *Journal of Psychotherapy and the Family, 3,* 79–96.

Kaslow, N. J., & Farber, E. (1995, August). *Working with severe psychopathology: Coping with therapist distress.* Paper presented at the 103rd annual convention of the American Psychological Association, New York.

Katz, J. F., & Hennessey, M. T. (1981). Which books are perceived as helpful in the training of psychotherapists? *Journal of Clinical Psychology, 37,* 505–506.

Kazak, A. E., & Noll, R. B. (2004). Child death from pediatric illness: Conceptualizing intervention from a family/systems and public health perspective. *Professional Psychology: Research and Practice, 35,* 219–226.

Keinan, G., Almagor, M., & Ben-Porath, Y. S. (1989). A reevaluation of the relationship between psychotherapeutic orientation and perceived personality characteristics. *Psychotherapy, 26,* 218–227.

Kelly, G. A. (1955). *The psychology of personal constructs.* New York: Norton.

Kiesler, D. J. (1966). Some myths of psychotherapy research and the search for a paradigm. *Psychological Bulletin, 65,* 110–136.

Kilburg, R. R., Nathan, E. N., & Thoreson, R. W. (Eds.). (1986). *Professionals in distress: Issues, syndromes, and solutions in psychology.* Washington, DC: American Psychological Association.

King, P. (1983). Identity crises: Splits or compromise—adaptive or maladaptive. In E. D. Joseph & D. Widlocher (Eds.), *The identity of the psychoanalyst.* New York: International Universities Press.

Kirschenbaum, H. (1979). *On becoming Carl Rogers.* New York: Delacorte.

Kleepies, P. M., Penk, W. E., & Forsyth, J. P. (1993). The stress of patient suicide behavior during clinical training: Incidence, impact, and recovery. *Professional Psychology: Research and Practice, 24,* 293–303.

Knapp, S., VandeCreek, L., & Phillips, A. (1993). Psychologists' worries about malpractice. *The Psychotherapy Bulletin, 28*(4), 46–47.

Koocher, G. P. (1999, June). Of dreams and duty. *APA Monitor,* 25.

Koocher, G. P., Norcross, J. C., & Hill, S. S. (Eds.). (2005). *Psychologists' desk reference* (2nd ed.). New York: Oxford University Press.

Kottler, J. A. (1986). *On being a therapist.* San Francisco: Jossey-Bass.

Kottler, J. A. (1993). *On being a therapist* (2nd ed.). San Francisco: Jossey-Bass.

Kottler, J. A. (1999). *The therapist's workbook.* San Francisco: Jossey-Bass.

Kottler, J. A. (2000). *Doing good: Passion and commitment for helping others.* New York: Brunner-Routledge.

Kottler, J. A., & Carlson, J. (Eds.). (2005). *The client who changed me: Stories of therapist personal transformation.* New York: Routledge.

Kramen-Kahn, B., & Hansen, N. D. (1998). Rafting the rapids: Occupational hazards, rewards, and coping strategies of psychotherapists. *Professional Psychology: Research and Practice, 29,* 130–134.

Lamb, D. H., Catanzaro, S. J., & Moorman, A. S. (2003). Psychologists reflect on their sexual relationships with clients, supervisees, and students: Occurrence, impact, rationales, and collegial intervention. *Professional Psychology: Research and Practice, 34,* 102–107.

Landon, B. E., Reschovsky, J., & Blumenthal, D. (2003). Changes in career satisfaction among primary care and specialist physicians, 1997–2001. *Journal of the American Medical Association, 289,* 442–449.

Lasky, R. (2005). The training analysis in the mainstream Freudian model. In J. D. Geller, J. C. Norcross, & D. E. Orlinsky (Eds.), *The psychotherapist's own psychotherapy.* New York: Oxford University Press.

Lazarus, A. A. (2000). Multimodal replenishment. *Professional Psychology: Research and Practice, 31,* 93–94.

Lazarus, A. A., & Zur, O. (Eds.). (2002). *Dual relationships and psychotherapy.* New York: Springer.

Leighton, S. L., & Royce, A. K. (1984). Spiritual self-care: That which replenishes the spirit battles burnout. *Family and Community Psychiatry, 6,* 44–56.

Leiter, M. P., & Maslach, C. (2005). *Banishing burnout: Six strategies for improving your relationship with work* San Francisco: Jossey-Bass.

Lewis, B. J. (2004, Spring). When the licensing board comes a'calling: Managing the stress of licensing board investigations. *The Independent Practitioner*, 121–124.

Lewis, C. S. (1942). *The screwtape letters.* New York: Harper.

Lewis, G. J., Greenburg, S. L., & Hatch, D. B. (1988). Peer consultation groups for psychologists in private practice: A national survey. *Professional Psychology: Research and Practice, 19*, 81–86.

Linehan, M. M. (1993). *Cognitive-behavioral treatment of borderline personality disorder.* New York: Guilford Press.

Little, L., & Hamby, S. L. (1996). Impact of a clinician's sexual abuse history, gender and theoretical orientation on treatment issues related to childhood sexual abuse. *Professional Psychology: Research and Practice, 27*, 617–625.

Lowe, W., Jr. (2005). Four ways to be older and better. *Psychotherapy Networker, 29*, 55.

Lyall, A. (1989). The prevention and treatment of professional burnout. In D. T. Wessells et al. (Eds.), *Professional burnout in medicine and the helping professions.* New York: Haworth.

Macran, S., & Shapiro, D. (1998). The role of personal therapy for therapists: A review. *British Journal of Medical Psychology, 71*, 13–25.

Mahoney, M. J. (1991). *Human change processes: The scientific foundations of psychotherapy.* New York: Basic Books.

Mahoney, M. J. (1997). Psychotherapist's personal problems and self-care patterns. *Professional Psychology: Research and Practice, 28*, 14–16.

Mahoney, M. J. (2003). *Constructive psychotherapy: A practical guide.* New York: Guilford Press.

Mahrer, A. R. (2000). How to use psychotherapy on, for, and by oneself. *Professional Psychology: Research and Practice, 31*, 226–229.

Maier, G. J., & Van Rybroek, G. J. (1995). Managing countertransference reactions to aggressive patients. In B. S. Eichelman & A. C. Hartwig (Eds.), *Patient violence and the clinician* (pp. 73–104). Washington, DC: American Psychiatric Press.

Margison, F. R. (1987). Stress in psychiatrists. In R. Payne & J. Firth-Coyens (Eds.), *Stress in health professions.* New York: Wiley.

Martin, R. A. (2001). Humor, laughter, and physical health: Methodological issues and research findings. *Psychological Bulletin, 127*, 504–519.

Maslach, C., & Goldberg, J. (1998). Prevention of burnout: New perspectives. *Applied and Preventive Psychology, 7*, 63–74.

Maslow, A. H. (1971). *The farther reaches of human nature.* New York: Viking.

Matthews, D. A., McCullough, M. E., Larson, D. B., Koenig, H. G., Swyers, J. P., & Milano, M. G. (1998). Religious commitment and health: A review of the research and implications for family medicine. *Archives of Family Medicine, 7*, 118–124.

McCollum, E. (1998). Restorying our roles: Preventing burnout through collaboration. *Psychotherapy Networker, 22*, 69.

Medeiros, M. E., & Prochaska, J. O. (1988). Coping strategies that psychotherapists use in working with stressful clients. *Professional Psychology: Research and Practice, 19,* 112–114.

Menninger, W. W. (1991). Patient suicide and its impact on the psychotherapist. *Bulletin of the Menninger Clinic, 55,* 216–227.

Miller, L. (1998). Our own medicine: Traumatized psychotherapists and the stresses of doing therapy. *Psychotherapy, 35,* 137–149.

Moore, T. (1992). *Care of the soul: A guide for cultivating depth and sacredness in everyday life.* New York: HarperCollins.

Morin, C. M., et al. (1999). Nonpharmacologic treatment of chronic insomnia: An American Academy of Sleep Medicine Review. *Sleep, 22,* 1134–1156.

Moyer, C. A., Rounds, J., & Hannum, J. W. (2004). A meta-analysis of massage therapy research. *Psychological Bulletin, 130,* 3–18.

Munsey, C. (2006, November). Questions of balance: An APA survey finds a lack of attention to self-care among training programs. *Graduate Psychology,* 37–39.

Murphy, B. C., & Dillon, C. (2002). *Interviewing in action: Process and practice* (2nd ed.). Pacific Grove, CA: Wadsworth.

Murphy, J. W., & Pardeck, J. T. (1986). The "burnout syndrome" and management style. *Clinical Supervisor, 4,* 35–44.

Murstein, B. I., & Mink, D. (2004). Do psychotherapists have better marriages than nonpsychotherapists? Do therapeutic skills and experience relate to marriage adjustment? *Psychotherapy, 41,* 292–300.

Myers, D. G. (1993). *The pursuit of happiness.* New York: Avon.

Myers, D. G. (2000). The funds, friends, and faith of happy people. *American Psychologist, 55,* 55–67.

Nash, J., Norcross, J. C., & Prochaska, J. O. (1984). Satisfactions and stresses of independent practice. *Psychotherapy in Private Practice, 2,* 39–48.

Neumann, D. A., & Gamble, S. J. (1995). Issues in the professional development of psychotherapists: Countertransference and vicarious traumatization in the new trauma therapist. *Psychotherapy, 32,* 341–347.

Nezu, A. M., Nezu, C. M., & Blissett, S. E. (1988). Sense of humor as a moderator of the relation between stressful events and psychological distress: A prospective analysis. *Journal of Personality and Social Psychology, 54,* 520–525.

Norcross, J. C. (1988). The exclusivity myth and the equifinality principle in psychotherapy. *Journal of Integrative and Eclectic Psychotherapy, 7,* 415–421.

Norcross, J. C. (2000). Psychotherapist self-care: Practitioner-tested, research-informed strategies. *Professional Psychology: Research and Practice, 31,* 710–713.

Norcross, J. C. (Ed.). (2002). *Psychotherapy relationships that work.* New York: Oxford University Press.

Norcross, J. C. (2005a). Lose not our moorings: Commentary on McWilliams. *Psychotherapy, 42,* 152–155.

Norcross, J. C. (2005b). The psychotherapist's own psychotherapy: Educating and developing psychologists. *American Psychologist, 60,* 840–850.

Norcross, J. C. (2006). Personal integration: An N of 1 study. *Journal of Psychotherapy Integration, 16,* 59–72.

Norcross, J. C., & Aboyoun, D. C. (1994). Self-change experiences of psychotherapists. In T. M. Brinthaupt & R. P. Lipka (Eds.), *Changing the self*. Albany: State University of New York Press.

Norcross, J. C., & Connor, K. A. (2005). Psychotherapists entering personal therapy: Their primary reasons and presenting problems. In J. D. Geller, J. C. Norcross, & D. E. Orlinsky (Eds.), *The psychotherapist's own psychotherapy*. New York: Oxford University Press.

Norcross, J. C., Dryden, W., & DeMichele, J. T. (1992). British clinical psychologists and personal therapy: What's good for the goose? *Clinical Psychology Forum, 44,* 29–33.

Norcross, J. C., & Goldfried, M. R. (Eds.). (2005). *Handbook of psychotherapy integration* (2nd ed.). New York: Oxford University Press.

Norcross, J. C., & Grunebaum, H. (2005). The selection and characteristics of therapists' psychotherapists: A research synthesis. In J. D. Geller, J. C. Norcross, & D. E. Orlinsky (Eds.), *The psychotherapist's own psychotherapy*. New York: Oxford University Press.

Norcross, J. C., & Guy, J. D. (1989). The prevalence and parameters of personal therapy in the United States. In J. D. Geller, J. C. Norcross, & D. E. Orlinsky (Eds.), *The psychotherapist's own psychotherapy*. New York: Oxford University Press.

Norcross, J. C., & Guy, J. D. (2005). Ten therapists: The process of becoming and being. In W. Dryden & L. Spurling (Eds.), *On becoming a psychotherapist* (pp. 215–239). London: Routledge.

Norcross, J. C., Karg, R., & Prochaska, J. O. (1997). Clinical psychologists and managed care: Some data from the Division 12 membership. *The Clinical Psychologist, 50*(1), 4–8.

Norcross, J. C., Karpiak, C. P., & Santoro, S. O. (2005). Clinical psychologists across the years: The Division of Clinical Psychology from 1960 to 2003. *Journal of Clinical Psychology, 61,* 1467–1483.

Norcross, J. C., & Knight, B. G. (2000). Psychotherapy and aging in the 21st century: Integrative themes. In S. H. Qualls & N. Abeles (Eds.), *Psychology and the aging revolution*. Washington, DC: American Psychological Association.

Norcross, J. C., & Lambert, M. J. (2005). The therapy relationship. In J. C. Norcross, L. E. Beutler, & R. F. Levant (Eds.), *Evidence-based practices in mental health: Debate and dialogue on the fundamental questions*. Washington, DC: American Psychological Association.

Norcross, J. C., & Prochaska, J. O. (1983). Psychotherapists in independent practice: Some findings and issues. *Professional Psychology: Research and Practice, 14,* 869–881.

Norcross, J. C., & Prochaska, J. O. (1986a). Psychotherapist heal thyself I: The psychological distress and self-change of psychologists, counselors, and laypersons. *Psychotherapy, 23,* 102–114.

Norcross, J. C., & Prochaska, J. O. (1986b). Psychotherapist heal thyself II: The self-initiated therapy-facilitated change of psychological distress. *Psychotherapy, 23,* 345–356.

Norcross, J. C., Prochaska, J. O., & DiClemente, C. C. (1986). Self-change of psychological distress: Laypersons' vs. psychologists' coping strategies. *Journal of Clinical Psychology, 42,* 834–840.

Norcross, J. C., Prochaska, J. O., & Hambrecht, M. (1991). Treating ourselves vs.

treating our clients: A replication with alcohol abuse. *Journal of Substance Abuse, 3*, 123–129.

Norcross, J. C., Strausser, D. J., & Faltus, F. J. (1988). The therapist's therapist. *American Journal of Psychotherapy, 42*, 53–66.

Norcross, J. C., Strausser-Kirtland, D. J., & Missar, C. D. (1988). The processes and outcomes of psychotherapists' personal treatment experiences. *Psychotherapy, 25*, 36–43.

O'Connor, M. F. (2001). On the etiology and effective management of professional distress and impairment among psychologists. *Professional Psychology: Research and Practice, 32*, 345–350.

O'Donnell, B. (1995, Spring). Dangerous work. *Conversations on Jesuit Higher Education, 7*, 3.

Okun, M. A., & Stock, W. A. (1987). Correlates and components of subjective well-being among the elderly. *Journal of Applied Gerontology, 6*, 95–112.

Orlinsky, D. E. (2005). Becoming and being a psychotherapist: A psychodynamic memoir and meditation. *Journal of Clinical Psychology: In Session, 61*, 999–1007.

Orlinsky, D. E., & Howard, K. I. (1977). The therapist's experience of psychotherapy. In A. S. Gurman & A. M. Razin (Eds.), *Effective psychotherapy: A handbook of research*. New York: Pergamon.

Orlinsky, D. E., Norcross, J. C., Rønnestad, M. H., & Wiseman, H. (2005). Outcomes and impacts of psychotherapists' personal therapy: A research review. In J. D. Geller, J. C. Norcross, & D. E. Orlinsky (Eds.), *The psychotherapist's own psychotherapy*. New York: Oxford University Press.

Orlinsky, D. E., & Rønnestad, M. H. (2005). *How psychotherapists develop: A study of therapeutic work and professional growth*. Washington, DC: American Psychological Association.

Overholser, J. C., & Fine, M. A. (1990). Defining boundaries of professional competence. *Professional Psychology: Research and Practice, 21*, 462–469.

Palmer, P. J. (2000). *Let your life speak: Listening for the voice of vocation*. San Francisco: Jossey-Bass.

Paluszny, M., & Pozanski, E. (1971). Reactions of patients during pregnancy of the psychotherapist. *Psychiatric Opinion, 13*, 20–25.

Parrish, M. M., & Quinn, P. (1999). Laughing your way to peace of mind: How a little humor helps caregivers survive. *Clinical and Social Work Journal, 27*, 203–211.

Pearlman, L. A., & Saakvitne, K. W. (1995). *Trauma and the therapist: Countertransference and vicarious traumatization in psychotherapy with incest survivors*. New York: Norton.

Pearson, J. E. (1986). The definition and measurement of social support. *Journal of Counseling and Development, 64*, 390–395.

Penley, J. A., Tomoka, J., & Wiebe, J. S. (2002). The association of coping to physical and psychological outcomes: A meta-analytic review. *Journal of Behavioral Medicine, 25*, 551–603.

Penzer, W. N. (1984). The psychopathology of the psychotherapist. *Psychotherapy in Private Practice, 2*(2), 51–59.

Perlman, B., & Hartman, E. A. (1982). Burnout: Summary and future research. *Human Relations, 35*, 283–305.

Persi, J. (1992). Top gun games: When therapists compete. *Transactional Analysis Journal, 22,* 144–152.

Phelps, R., Eisman, E. J., & Kohout, J. (1998). Psychological practice and managed care: Results of the CAPP Practitioner Survey. *Professional Psychology: Research and Practice, 32,* 597–606.

Piercy, F. P., & Wetchler, J. L. (1987). Family–work interfaces of psychotherapists. *Journal of Psychotherapy and the Family, 3,* 17–32.

Pines, A. M., & Maslach, C. (1978). Characteristics of staff burnout in mental health settings. *Hospital and Community Psychiatry, 29,* 233–237.

Pirsig, R. (1974). *Zen and the art of motorcycle maintenance.* New York: Morrow.

Pomerantz, A. M., & Handelsman, M. H. (2004). Informed consent revisited: An updated written question format. *Professional Psychology: Research and Practice, 35,* 201–205.

Pope, K. S. (1991). Dual relationships in psychotherapy. *Ethics and Behavior, 1,* 21–34.

Pope, K. S. (1993). Licensing disciplinary actions for psychologists who have been sexually involved with a client. *Professional Psychology: Research and Practice, 24,* 374–377.

Pope, K. S., & Bouhoutsos, J. C. (1986). *Sexual intimacy between therapists and patients.* New York: Praeger.

Pope, K. S., Sonne, J. L., & Greene, B. (2006). *What therapists don't talk about and why: Understanding taboos that hurt us and our clients.* Washington, DC: American Psychological Association.

Pope, K. S., Sonne, J. L., & Holroyd, J. (1993). *Sexual feelings in psychotherapy.* Washington, DC: American Psychological Association.

Pope, K. S., & Tabachnick, B. G. (1993). Therapists' anger, hate, fear, and sexual feelings: National survey of therapist responses, client characteristics, critical events, formal complaints, and training. *Professional Psychology: Research and Practice, 24,* 142–152.

Pope, K. S., Tabachnick, B. G., & Keith-Spiegel, P. (1987). Ethics of practice: The beliefs and behaviors of psychologists as therapists. *American Psychologist, 42,* 993–1006.

Pope, K. S., Tabachnick, B. G., & Keith-Spiegel, P. (1988). Good and poor practices in psychotherapy: National survey of beliefs of psychologists. *Professional Psychology: Research and Practice, 19,* 547–552.

Pope, K. S., & Vasquez, M. J. T. (2005). *How to survive and thrive as a therapist: Information, ideas, and resources for psychologists in practice.* Washington, DC: American Psychological Association.

Poulin, J. E., & Walter, C. A. (1993). Social worker burnout: A longitudinal study. *Social Work Research and Abstracts, 29,* 5–11.

Powell, L. H., Shahabi, L., & Thoreson, C. E. (2003). Religion and spirituality: Linkages to physical health. *American Psychologist, 58,* 36–52.

Prochaska, J. O., & Norcross, J. C. (1983). Psychotherapists' perspectives on treating themselves and their clients for psychic distress. *Professional Psychology: Research and Practice, 14,* 642–655.

Prochaska, J. O., Norcross, J. C., & DiClemente, C. C. (1995). *Changing for good.* New York: Avon.

Psychotherapy Finances. (2004) Home page. Retrieved 2004 from *www.psyfin.com.*

Psychotherapy Networker. (2004). Special feature: The citizen-therapist. *Psychotherapy Networker, 28*(6), 32–50.

Purcell, R., Powell, M. B., & Mullen, P. E. (2005). Clients who stalk psychologists: Prevalence, methods, and motives. *Professional Psychology: Research and Practice, 36,* 537–543.

Radeke, J. T., & Mahoney, M. J. (2000). Comparing the personal lives of psychotherapists and research psychologists. *Professional Psychology: Research and Practice, 31,* 82–84.

Raider, M. C. (1989). Burnout in children's agencies: A clinician's perspective. *Residential Treatment for Children and Youth, 6,* 43–51.

Ragan, C., Malony, H. N., & Beit-Hallahmi, B. (1980). Psychologists and religion: Professional factors and personal belief. *Review of Religious Research, 21,* 208–217.

Rappoport, P. S. (1983). *Value for value psychotherapy: The economic and therapeutic barter.* New York: Praeger.

Raquepaw, J. M., & Miller, R. S. (1989). Psychotherapist burnout: A componential analysis. *Professional Psychology: Research and Practice, 20,* 32–36.

Rippere, V., & Williams, R. (Eds.). (1985). *Wounded healers: Mental health workers' experiences of depression.* New York: Wiley.

Romans, J. S., Hays, J. R., & White, T. K. (1996). Stalking and related behaviors experienced by counseling center staff members from current or former clients. *Professional Psychology: Research and Practice, 27,* 595–599.

Rønnestad, M. H., & Skovholt, T. M. (2001). Learning arenas for professional development: Retrospective accounts of senior psychotherapists. *Professional Psychology: Research and Practice, 32,* 181–187.

Rosenbaum, R. (1999). *Zen and the heart of psychotherapy.* New York: Brunner/ Mazel.

Rothbaum, P. A., Bernstein, D. M., Haller, O., Phelps, R., & Kohout, J. (1998). New Jersey psychologists' report on managed mental health care. *Professional Psychology: Research and Practice, 29,* 37–42.

Rothenberg, A. (1988). *The creative process of psychotherapy.* New York: Norton.

Royak-Schaler, R., & Feldman, R. H. L. (1984). Health behaviors of psychotherapists. *Journal of Clinical Psychology, 40,* 705–710.

Rupert, P. A., & Baird, K. A. (2004). Managed care and the independent practice of psychology. *Professional Psychology: Research and Practice, 35,* 185–193.

Rupert, P. A., & Kent, J. S. (2007). Gender and work setting differences in career-sustaining behaviors and burnout among professional psychologists. *Professional Psychology: Research and Practice, 38,* 88–96.

Ryan, K. (1999). Self-help for the helpers: Preventing vicarious traumatization. In N. B. Webb (Ed.), *Play therapy with children in crisis* (2nd ed., pp. 471–491). New York: Guilford Press.

Sacks, O. W. (1985). *The man who mistook his wife for a hat and other clinical tales.* New York: Summit.

Sapienza, B. G., & Bugental, J. F. T. (2000). Keeping our instruments finely tuned: An existential–humanistic perspective. *Professional Psychology: Research and Practice, 31,* 458–460.

Schaufeli, W. B., Maslach, C., & Marek, T. (Eds.). (1993). *Professional burnout: Recent developments in theory and research.* Washington, DC: Taylor & Francis.

Schneider, K. J. (2004). *Rediscovery of awe.* St. Paul, MN: Paragon House.

Schoenfeld, L. S., Hatch, J. P., & Gonzalez, J. M. (2001). Responses of psychologists to complaints filed against them with a state licensing board. *Professional Psychology: Research and Practice, 5,* 491-495.

Schroder, T. A., & Davis, J. D. (2004). Therapists' experience of difficulty in practice. *Psychotherapy research, 14,* 328-345.

Schwartz, H. J. (1987). Illness in the doctor: Implications for the psychoanalytic process. *Journal of the American Psychoanalytic Association, 35,* 657-692.

Schwartz, R. (2004). The larger self. *Psychotherapy Networker, 28,* 37-43.

Schwebel, M., & Coster, J. (1998). Well-functioning in professional psychologists: As program heads see it. *Professional Psychology: Research and Practice, 29,* 284-292.

Scott, C. D., & Hawk, J. (Eds.). (1986). *Heal thyself: The health of health care professionals.* New York: Brunner/Mazel.

Shafranske, E. P., & Malony, H. N. (1990). Clinical psychologists' religious and spiritual orientations and their practice of psychotherapy. *Psychotherapy, 27,* 72-78.

Sharkin, B. S., & Birky, I. (1992). Incidental encounters between therapists and their clients. *Professional Psychology: Research and Practice, 23,* 326-328.

Shaw, R. (2004). The embodied psychotherapist: An exploration of the therapists' somatic phenomena within the therapeutic encounter. *Psychotherapy Research, 14,* 271-288.

Sherman, M. D., & Thelen, M. H. (1998). Distress and professional impairment among psychologists in clinical practice. *Professional Psychology: Research and Practice, 29,* 79-85.

Shoyer, B. G. (February, 1999). Psychotherapist self-care: Beliefs, practices, and outcomes. *Dissertation Abstracts International: Section B, 59,* 4485.

Skorupa, J. K., & Agresti, A. A. (1993). Ethical beliefs about burnout and continued professional practice. *Professional Psychology: Research and Practice, 24,* 281-285.

Skovholt, T. M., & Jennings, L. (2004). *Master therapists: Exploring expertise in therapy and counseling.* New York: Allyn & Bacon.

Slimp, P. A., & Burian, B. K. (1994). Multiple role relationships during internship: Consequences and recommendations. *Professional Psychology, 25,* 39-45.

Sloan, D. M., & Marx, B. P. (2004). Taking pen to hand: Evaluating theories underlying the written disclosure paradigm. *Clinical Psychology: Science and Practice, 11,* 121-137.

Sloboda, J. (1999). Music—where cognition and emotion meet. *Psychologist, 12,* 450-455.

Smith, D. P., & Orlinsky, D. E. (2004). Religion and spiritual experience among psychotherapists. *Psychotherapy, 41,* 144-151.

Smith, J., Staudinger, U. M., & Baltes, P. B. (1994). Occupational settings facilitating wisdom-related knowledge: The sample case of clinical psychologists. *Journal of Consulting and Clinical Psychology, 62,* 989-999.

Smith, M. T., et al. (2002). Comparative meta-analysis of pharmacotherapy and behavior therapy for persistent insomnia. *American Journal of Psychiatry, 159,* 5-11.

Snibbe, J. R., Radcliffe, T., Weisberger, C., Richards, M., & Kelly, J. (1989). Burnout among primary care physicians and mental health professionals in a managed health care setting. *Psychological Reports, 65,* 775–780.

Spiegel, P. B. (1990). Confidentiality endangered under some circumstances without special management. *Psychotherapy, 27,* 636–641.

Stake, J. E., & Oliver, J. (1991). Sexual contact and touching between therapist and client. *Professional Psychology: Research and Practice, 22,* 297–307.

Stathopoulou, G., Powers, M. B., Berry, A. C., Smits, J. A. J., & Otto, M. W. (2006). Exercise interventions for mental health: A quantitative and qualitative review. *Clinical Psychology: Science and Practice, 13,* 179–193.

Sternlieb, J. L. (2005, January). Balint—an underutilized tool. *The Pennsylvania Psychologist Update,* 8–9.

Stevanovic, P., & Rupert, P. A. (2004). Career-sustaining behaviors, satisfactions, and stresses of professional psychologists. *Psychotherapy, 41,* 301–309.

Stricker, G. (1995). Comment: Confessions of a reformed psychodynamicist. *Journal of Psychotherapy Integration, 5,* 266–267.

Sullivan, T., Martin, W. L., Jr., & Handelsman, M. M. (1993). Practical benefits of an informed consent procedure: An empirical investigation. *Journal of Clinical Psychology, 54,* 115–120.

Sussman, M. B. (Ed.). (1995). *A perilous calling: The hazards of psychotherapy practice.* New York: Wiley.

Tabachnick, B. G., Keith-Spiegel, P., & Pope, K. S. (1991). Ethics of teaching. *American Psychologist, 46,* 506–515.

Tamura, L. J., Guy, J. D., Brady, J. L., & Grace, C. (1994). Maintaining confidentiality, avoiding burnout and psychotherapists' needs for inclusion: A national survey. *Psychotherapy in Private Practice, 13,* 1–17.

Taylor, S. W., Klein, L. C., Lewis, B. P., Gruenewald, T. L., Gurung, R. A. R., & Updegraff, J. A. (2000). Female response to stress: Tend and befriend, not fight or flight. *Psychological Review, 107,* 411–429.

Thoreau, H. D. (1854). *Walden.* Boston: Ticknor & Fields.

Thoreson, R. W., Budd, F. C., & Krauskopf, C. J. (1986). Alcoholism among psychologists: Factors in relapse and recovery. *Professional Psychology: Research and Practice, 17,* 497–503.

Thoreson, R. W., Miller, M., & Krauskopf, C. J. (1989). The distressed psychologist: Prevalence and treatment considerations. *Professional Psychology: Research and Practice, 20,* 153–158.

Thorne, B. (1988). The blessing and curse of empathy. In W. Dryden & L. Spurling (Eds.), *On becoming a psychotherapist.* London: Croom Helm.

Tieman, P. A. (1987). The satisfactions and stresses of pastoral psychotherapy. *Journal of Pastoral Psychotherapy, 1,* 39–49.

Tryon, G. S. (1983). The pleasures and displeasures of full-time private practice. *The Clinical Psychologist, 36,* 45–48.

Tryon, G. S., & Winograd, G. (2002). Goal consensus and collaboration. In J. C. Norcross (Ed.), *Psychotherapy relationships that work.* New York: Oxford University Press.

Turner, J. A., Edwards, L. M., Eicken, I. M., Yokoyama, K., Castro, J. R., Tran, A. N., et al. (2005). Intern self-care: An exploratory study into strategy use and effectiveness. *Professional Psychology: Research and Practice, 36,* 674–680.

Wachtel, P. L. (1977). *Psychoanalysis and behavior therapy: Toward an integration.* New York: Basic Books.

Wahl, W. K., Guy, J. D., & Brown, C. K. (1993). Conducting psychotherapy: Impact upon the therapist's marital relationship. *Psychotherapy in Private Practice, 12,* 57–60.

Walfish, S., Moritz, J. L., & Stenmark, D. E. (1991). A longitudinal study of the career satisfaction of clinical psychologists. *Professional Psychology: Research and Practice, 22,* 253–255.

Walsh, S., & Cormack, M. (1994). "Do as we say but not as we do": Organizational, professional and personal barriers to the receipt of support at work. *Clinical Psychology and Psychotherapy, 1,* 101–110.

Wampold, B. E. (2001). *The great psychotherapy debate: Models, methods, and findings.* Mahwah, NJ: Erlbaum.

Wampold, B. E., & Brown, G. S. (2005). Estimating variability in outcomes attributable to therapists: A naturalistic study of outcomes in managed care. *Journal of Consulting and Clinical Psychology, 73,* 914–923.

Warner, S. L. (1991). Humor: A coping response for student nurses. *Archives of Psychiatric Nursing, 5,* 10–16.

Weiss, L. (2004). *Therapist's guide to self-care.* New York: Brunner–Routledge.

Weiss, L., & Weiss, B. W. (1992). Personal reminiscences of a psychologist married couple on changing perspectives in 20 years of professional psychology. *Professional Psychology: Research and Practice, 23,* 349–352.

Wetchler, J., & Piercy, F. P. (1986). The marital and family life of the family therapist: Stressors and enhancers. *American Journal of Family Therapy, 14,* 99–108.

Whitaker, C. A., & Bumberry, W. M. (1988). *Dancing with the family: A symbolic experiential approach.* New York: Brunner/Mazel.

White, M. (1997). *Narratives of therapists' lives.* Adelaide, South Australia: Dulwich Centre Publications.

Wierzbicki, M., & Pekarik, G. (1993). A meta-analysis of psychotherapy dropout. *Professional Psychology: Research and Practice, 24,* 190–195.

Wilbert, J. R., & Fulero, S. M. (1988). Impact of malpractice litigation on professional psychology. *Professional Psychology: Research and Practice, 19,* 379–382.

Will, O. A. (1979). Comments on the professional life of the psychotherapist. *Contemporary Psychoanalysis, 15,* 560–575.

Williams-Nickelson, C. (2006). Balanced living through self-care. In J. Worell & C. D. Goodheart (Eds.), *Handbook of girls' and women's psychological health.* New York: Oxford University Press.

Winnicott, D. W. (1958). *Through pediatrics to psychoanalysis.* London: Tavistock Publications.

Wogan, M., & Norcross, J. C. (1985). Dimensions of psychotherapeutic skills and techniques: Empirical identification, therapist correlates, and predictive utility. *Psychotherapy, 22,* 63–74.

Wolfe, J. L. (2000). A vacation from musterbation. *Professional Psychology: Research and Practice, 31,* 581–583.

Wood, B., Klein, S., Cross, H. J., Lammers, C. J., & Elliot, J. K. (1985). Impaired practitioners: Psychologists' opinions about prevalence, and proposals for intervention. *Professional Psychology: Research and Practice, 16,* 843–850.

Wykes, T., & Whittington, R. (1991). Coping strategies used by staff following assault by a patient: An exploratory study. *Work and Stress, 5,* 37–48.

Yager, J., & Borus, J. F. (1990). A survival guide for psychiatric residency training directors. *Academic Psychiatry, 14,* 180–187.

Yalom, I. D. (1975). *The theory and practice of group psychotherapy.* New York: Basic Books.

Yalom, I. D. (2002). *The gift of therapy.* New York: HarperCollins.

Zur, O. (1993). Avoiding the hazards of your profession. *The California Psychologist, 26,* 16.

Index